HOW TO LOOK
Pretty Not Plastered

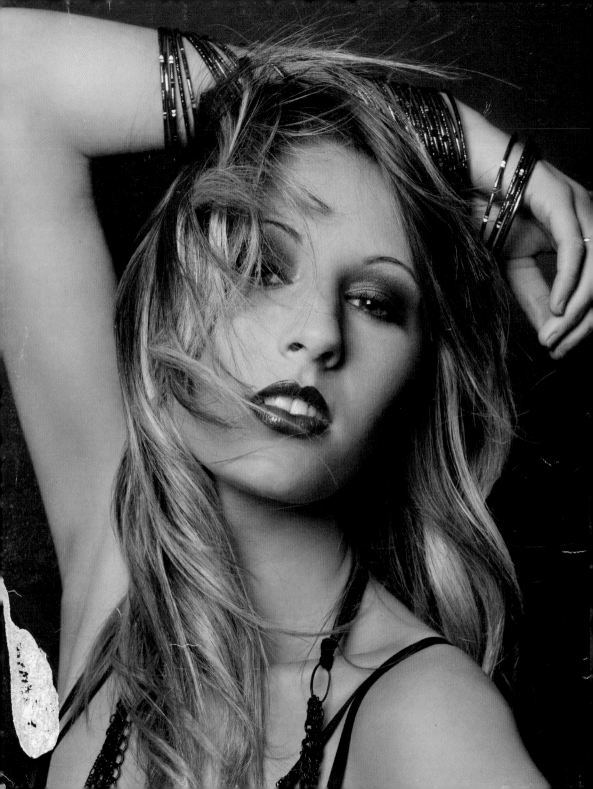

HOW TO LOOK

Pretty Not Plastered

A step-by-step make-up guide to looking great!

Emily Rose

howtobooks

Published by How To Books Ltd
Spring Hill House, Spring Hill Road
Begbroke, Oxford OX5 1RX
United Kingdom
Tel: (01865) 375794
Fax: (01865) 379162
info@howtobooks.co.uk
www.howtobooks.co.uk

First published 2011

British Library Cataloguing in Publication Data
A catalogue record of this book is available from the British Library.

ISBN: 978 1 84528 475 6

Produced for How To Books by Deer Park Productions, Tavistock, Devon
Designed and typeset by Mousemat Design Ltd
Printed and bound in Spain by Graphy Cems

NOTE: The material contained in this book is set out in good faith for general guidance and no liability can be accepted for loss or expense incurred as a result of relying in particular circumstances on statements made in the book. Laws and regulations are complex and liable to change, and readers should check the current position with relevant authorities before making personal arrangements.

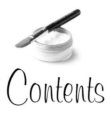

Contents

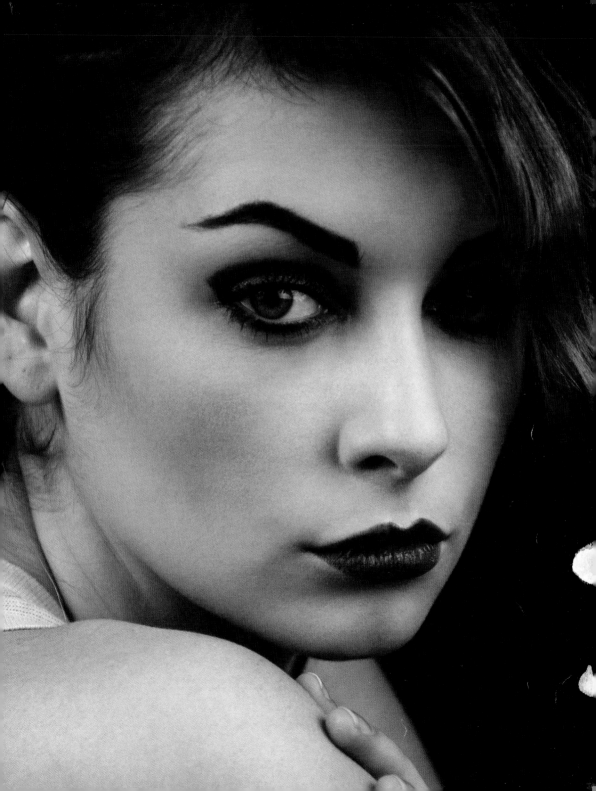

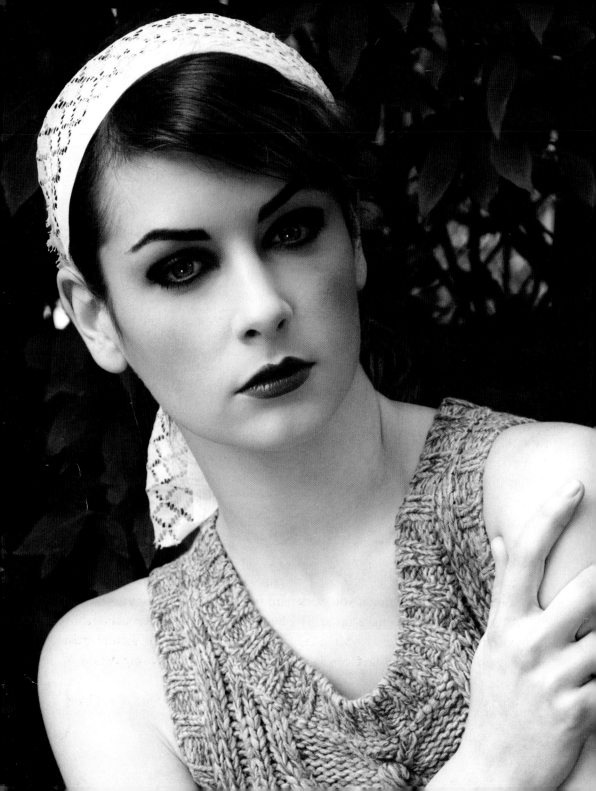

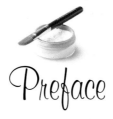

Preface

My passion for make-up reaches back into childhood, from the time I first began to 'paint'. Born into an artistic family, I soon discovered I had talent and have continued to nurture it to this day.

I began in art college, where I drew portrait after portrait. I wanted to create some work that was different from everyone else's, so I used my love of make-up and began experimenting with different products, teaching myself, and using the face as my blank canvas. I brought models into the college studio, created a fantastic make-up for them, styled their hair and clothes and photographed them for my portfolio. I knew instantly that this was where my passion lay – as a make-up artist.

After I left college I was lucky enough to meet a world-famous make-up artist and skincare specialist who inspired me to turn my dream into reality. When, at 20, I had my daughter Lara I became even more ambitious. I was determined to become a positive role model for her as she grows up. I wanted her to understand that you can achieve anything if you work hard for it and stay true to your beliefs.

After qualifying as a make-up artist I began sourcing work throughout the fashion, advertising, film and wedding industries, working alongside another artist to build up my knowledge and confidence. Eventually I achieved my dream of becoming a successful make-up artist.

I have written this book for young women, to teach you the art of applying perfect make-up and still looking like beautiful you.

I want to replace the myth of perfect images shown in magazines and advertisements and help you to create a look that's right for you, your skin, and – most importantly – your age. Most of all, I want to show you how to have fun with your make-up.

This is one of the best times of your life. You are young enough to wear the brightest, boldest colours and get away with it. Enjoy!

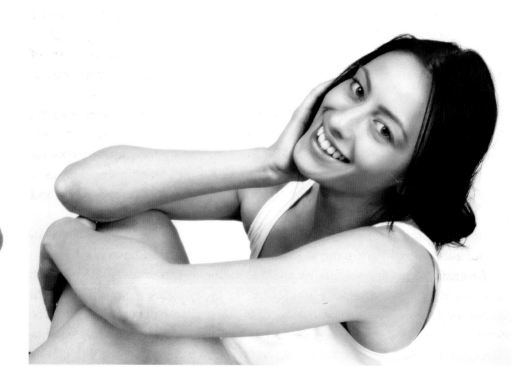

CHAPTER 1

Introduction

Real beauty & the myth of perfection

As modern technology becomes more advanced, so models and celebrities are helped to look even more flawless with the use of digital editing. But is this a positive development for teen girls?

Young girls are looking more adult than ever, as they aspire to the world of celebrities and fashion, seeking guidance from beautiful role models in the media. Everything screams make-up, and lots of it!

Girls relate to this seemingly perfect existence, because being a teen or young adult involves a lot of image consciousness – I know, I was one not too long ago. The fact is, nobody is perfect, and these clever Photoshop techniques encourage girls to believe that make-up alone is what makes women look flawless. It's just a clever marketing strategy. But it is my job to show you how it is really done, and that looking pretty isn't about being plastered in make-up.

In this book I want to teach you exactly how to achieve flawless make-up, without airbrushing! I am going to teach you what real beauty looks like.

Magazines are fabulous fun, we all love reading them and catching up on the latest gossip, trends and real-life articles, but please be aware that not everything you see or read is true. Magazines need to look exciting and current, and are therefore as full of stories as they are real life. Fashion magazines are designed to make us think: 'Wow, I want to look like her!', because that makes them sell! How many times have you seen a gorgeous dress or a pair of shoes in a magazine, maybe the latest lip gloss, and gone out to buy it? I know I have!

If there is one thing that I have learnt along my journey, it's that celebrities are just real people, like you or me. In the same way as actors play a part, many celebrities too adopt a particular character that suits the image they wish to promote to the media.

Photoshop techniques are carried out on almost every photo we see in the media. It is possible to retouch an image and completely transform a person's looks.

For example, you can:

- add or change the colour of make-up;
- boost the colour and texture of hair;
- make an imperfect complexion flawless;
- whiten and straighten teeth;
- whiten and widen eyes;
- make arms, legs and waists look slimmer;
- make breasts larger;
- remove imperfections;
- add a tan.

The list is endless!

In recent years there has been a lot of debate about the use of digitally enhanced images. This has resulted in magazines demanding that advertorial images identify where some digital enhancement has been used. For instance, in mascara advertisements where false lashes have been used to emphasise the product, you will often see included some small print at the bottom of the page which identifies this.

So, next time you think, 'I wish I looked like that', remember that it isn't always as real as you may be led to believe.

Be comfortable with who you are. Don't let spots, blemishes, scars or moles get you down; these characteristics are all part of the beautiful and individual people that we are. We tend to be critical of ourselves and worry about imperfections that other people might not even notice. Remember that confidence makes you glow, and inner and outer beauty work in harmony.

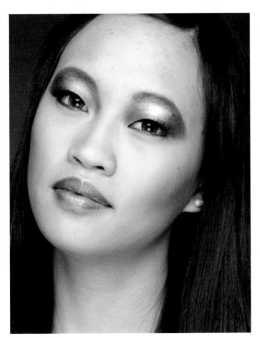 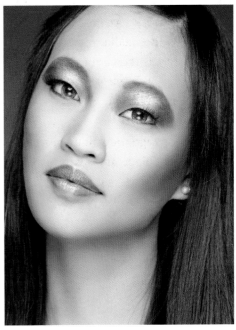

Look at these two images.

You will see immediately that the model looks more striking in the second image. However, it isn't just that the blemishes have been removed and the skin has been airbrushed. Look a little closer and you will notice that:

- the jaw line is squarer;
- the nose has been narrowed;
- any under eye darkness has been removed;
- the eyes have been brightened;
- the face has been slimmed;
- the lips have been narrowed.

These improvements are typical of those applied to any editorial image, and many are taken a lot further than this to enhance the beauty of the model.

In extreme cases faces and features are mirrored to ensure symmetry. It is said that the most beautiful faces are those that are the most symmetrical; the features are exactly the same on either side of the face. Creative people whose job is to enhance images go to great lengths to achieve this ideal; no wonder we see these images and wish we looked like the model staring back at us. In reality, it is very rare that people's faces are completely symmetrical.

In this book the vast majority of images have not been digitally enhanced to any great extent, so that everything you see in the book can be achieved purely through applying your make-up using the correct technique.

What is airbrushing?

We hear the word airbrushing an awful lot these days, particularly since the airbrush make-up has become so popular. When an image is digitally airbrushed, it means that the skin is completely perfected; it is smoothed over, lightened, brightened and given a glow.

Airbrush make-up is used for the same reason; the fine spray creates a completely smooth, even base that appears flawless.

A world full of make-up

Now, more than ever, one of the biggest trends is for natural beauty. Take it from me, though: looking beautiful while at the same time appearing to be wearing little – if any – make-up is a real art.

Make-up can completely transform a person, for better or worse, depending on how well it is applied. I often meet older women who are keen to have make-up lessons. Many tell me they wish their mum had known how to apply make-up properly so that they could have learnt the secrets as a teenager. So I am going to teach you those secrets in this book, so that one day perhaps you can pass on this valuable information to your own daughters, or to your friends.

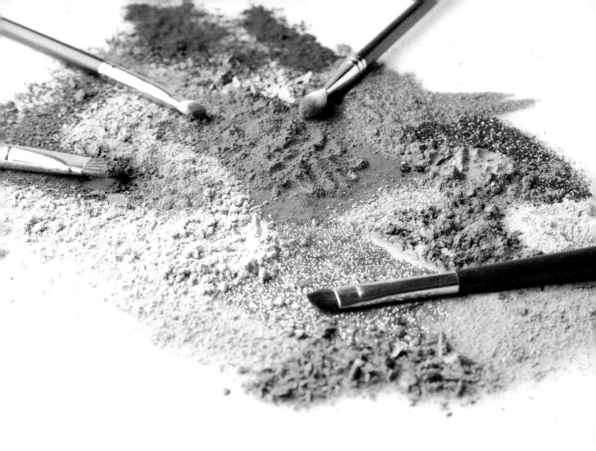

How to look pretty *not* plastered

Young women's make-up should be natural and reflect their age, but this doesn't mean it has to be invisible. I am well aware as a make-up artist that we don't always want to look as if we aren't wearing any make-up. On a night out we love smoky eyes, glitter, colour and fun! There is a lot of coverage in the media at the moment promoting natural make-up, but this doesn't mean it has to be plain. The point is, foundation is skin-coloured for a reason – it is designed to be invisible. Bright eye make-up and bright lipsticks on the other hand are designed to be noticed! Team the two ideas together and you will look pretty, and not plastered.

Your skin is at its best at this time of your life so it is important to look after it. Have fun with make-up and be unique. This is the perfect time to play with colour, especially for parties!

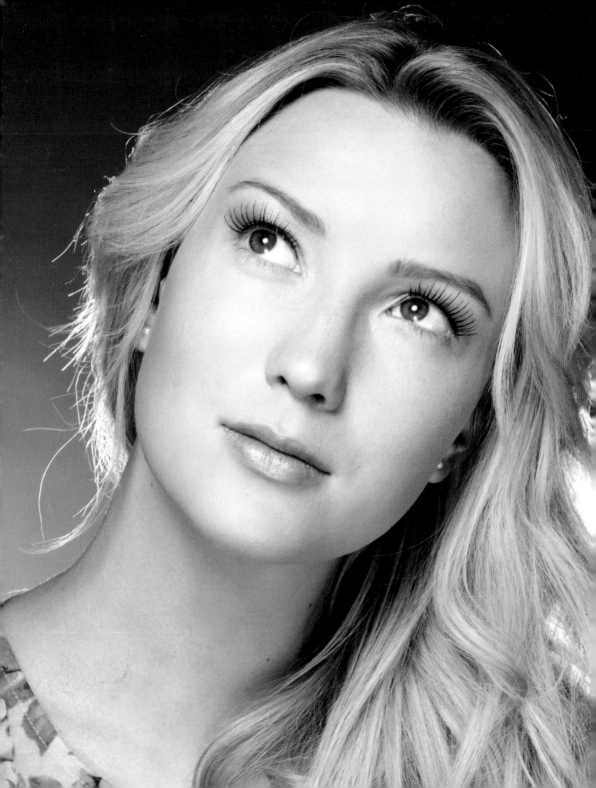

During the day, keep your make-up simple, natural and fresh-looking; all you really need is a good mascara, concealer to cover any blemishes, blusher to give you a healthy, radiant glow, and lip gloss.

Shimmery, metallic and iridescent colours look best on young girls, as they complement youthful, beautiful skin. Matt, dark colours tend to be less flattering because they can look heavy.

Avoid thick eyeliner drawn all the way around your eyes, especially in the daytime. It makes eyes look small, dark and much too heavy. If you like the effect of eyeliner, use an eyeshadow instead.

Remember, when you apply make-up, less is more. Too much looks fake, so apply it with a light touch.

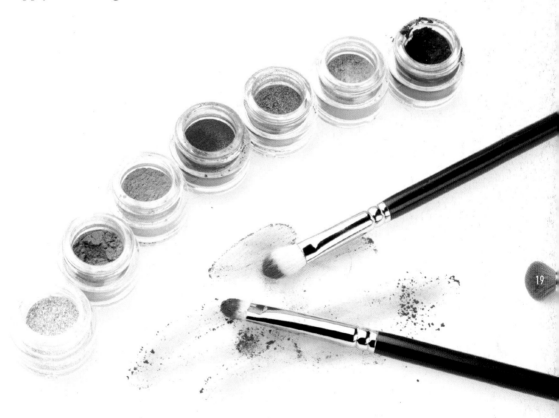

The first simple rule to pretty make-up is exactly that – keep it simple! Focus on one or two features only; never three, as this will look too made-up. See the examples below.

- Bright eyes; natural lips; natural, healthy cheeks;
- Bright eyes; bright lips; natural, healthy cheeks;
- Natural eyes; bright lips; natural, healthy cheeks;
- Natural eyes; natural lips; natural, healthy cheeks.

> **Top Tip:** Natural cheeks always look best unless you are creating a fashion or fancy dress look.

If you plaster make-up on to hide behind, you'll find it doesn't work. In fact people notice it, and you, more. Instead learn to love the way you look; if you do, others will too, and you'll be surprised how quickly you grow in confidence and settle into your own skin.

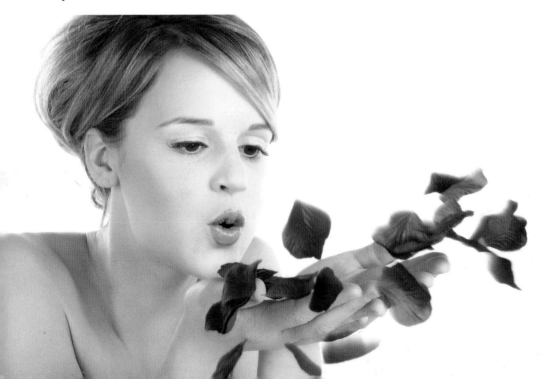

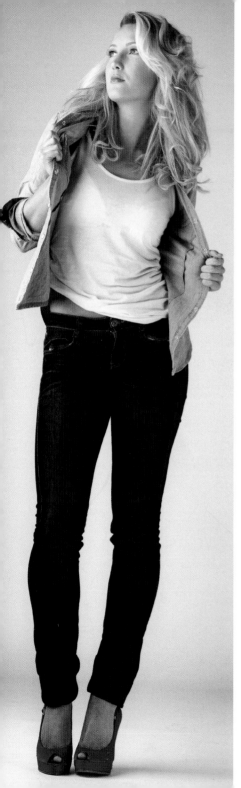

Have fun with your make-up

Enjoy experimenting with make-up and don't try to appear too grown-up, as this only looks false. Enjoy your youth; the ratio of young to older years is far too low!

When I was 14, I looked 14, walking around in big jumpers and jeans, with barely a scrape of make-up on my face. Today's young girls, in their fashionable clothes, high heels and make-up, often look much older than their years.

Yet, despite their passion for clothes and fashion, I am shocked at how few of them actually know how to apply their make-up properly. Orange faces and thick black eyeliner are some of the many mistakes I see.

Young girls, and even mature women, often don't realise that foundation isn't meant to change the colour of our skin or cover all of our blemishes; it's intended purely to even out our natural skin tone. Bronzer, not foundation, adds colour; concealer/camouflage covers.

I recently worked with a group of 14-year-old girls who were having a makeover and photo shoot party. These girls were very pretty and looked very mature indeed. In fact, as a mother myself, I felt justified in advising one of the girls to take off her enormously high heels because she looked too grown-up!

I decided to include a mini make-up lesson within the party to show the girls how to apply their make-up properly, at the same time

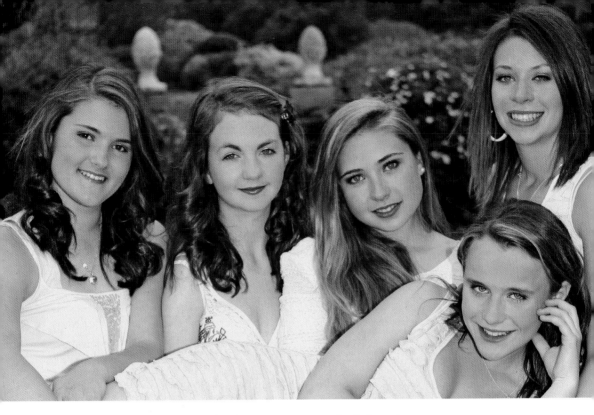

demonstrating the difference between teen and adult make-up.

All the girls were blessed with perfect, blemish-free skin. Nevertheless, one of them explained that she liked to wear a lot of foundation. Why? I asked. The answer was: pressure to appear perfect, from every airbrushed magazine photo, every catwalk model and every piece of commercial material that we see all around us.

I also discovered that very few girls actually understand the ingredients and chemicals that go into cosmetics and how they affect your skin. I realise that young, image-conscious girls suffering from acne and breakouts may not want to go without any make-up at all, but please be aware that clogging your pores further will only add to the problem. Teen skin is young and should be allowed to breathe. Natural skincare products are becoming a hot topic, but not many of these are directed at the teen market.

I want to show you how important it is to look after your skin, and how to keep it beautiful. Make-up should be used as a means of enhancing your natural glow, not to create a mask to hide behind.

Discover your unique style

Masking yourself in make-up does not increase confidence. I spoke to a young lady who had worn heavy eyeliner every day since she began wearing make-up. When I experimented by removing it, she lacked confidence because she wasn't used to being without it, with being her natural self. So, don't be afraid to experiment and don't be afraid of change. Fashion and beauty are about finding your own unique, individual style; this is what makes each one of us memorable.

Girls also need to understand not only how to apply their make-up but also the difference between adult and teen make-up application. One of the main reasons that teenage girls are looking more like young adults is because they are recreating the adult looks that they see on celebrities and in glossy magazines.

Make-up applied this way on young girls looks very overdone. Although girls may think they are creating a more mature look, in reality they simply look like teens with too much make-up on, trying to look older than they really are. Not only is this creating a false image, but they are projecting a false illusion of their age that can put them at risk.

You can look beautiful without looking over-made-up if you follow some simple make-up rules which I will show you in this book.

To be truly happy, you must be happy with yourself; when you are happy with yourself, you will sparkle! If you learn this lesson now, as a young woman, you will go a long way towards becoming a more confident person.

CHAPTER 2

Beautiful Skin

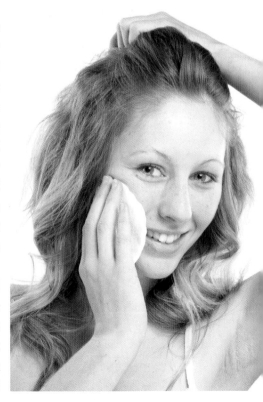

Look after your beautiful skin

As a teenager, your hormone levels will be forever changing as puberty begins and your body starts to develop. All of these hormonal changes have an effect on both your inner and outer self, which means that this is the most vital time to begin to take care of your body. It is extremely important to understand the characteristics of your own skin type, how to take care of it, and which products will benefit you. Make-up should do more than just even out your skin tone or add colour; it should be a truly nourishing cosmetic product.

I am a great advocate of natural products, which really boost and repair your skin. Choose your products wisely; although there are some cheap products on the market which may look good, this doesn't mean that they are necessarily good for your skin. Read the list of ingredients carefully. Many chain-store brands contain synthetic ingredients which clog the pores and don't allow your skin to breathe.

I believe that a foundation or skincare product should be as close to 100% natural as possible, in order to feed your skin and allow it to breathe. Many teens suffer from acne along with other skin conditions. They are also commonly affected by problems such as oily or very dry skin. It makes sense therefore to use a product that is designed specifically to help your particular problem. That way you will start the process of recovery, which can benefit you in adult life, leaving you with healthy, manageable skin.

I recently worked with an actress who had beautiful skin and was wearing barely any make-up. As I began applying her make-up for a film, she explained to me that as a teenager she had not worn any make-up at all because she suffered from severe acne. She had felt that if she wore make-up over her spots it would be too much, so she stopped wearing it altogether and used a cream prescribed by her doctor. Ten years on, her complexion is as near to perfect as it can be and she strongly believes that by leaving her skin to breathe, it began to repair itself.

Achieve healthy, glowing skin

We are constantly advised by health experts to 'drink plenty of water, eat well, sleep well, relax and exercise' – five pieces of advice that we all tend to put to one side as our busy lives become even busier. But stop, relax and consider the impact on your skin and well-being of ignoring such sensible suggestions. As clichéd as it may sound, these truly are the five main factors for gorgeous, glowing skin. After these comes a perfect make-up application.

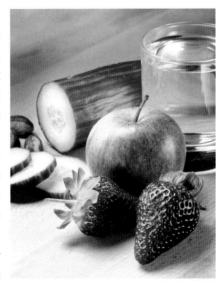

Dehydration is a number one factor for breakouts and dry, flaky skin. Although, as a

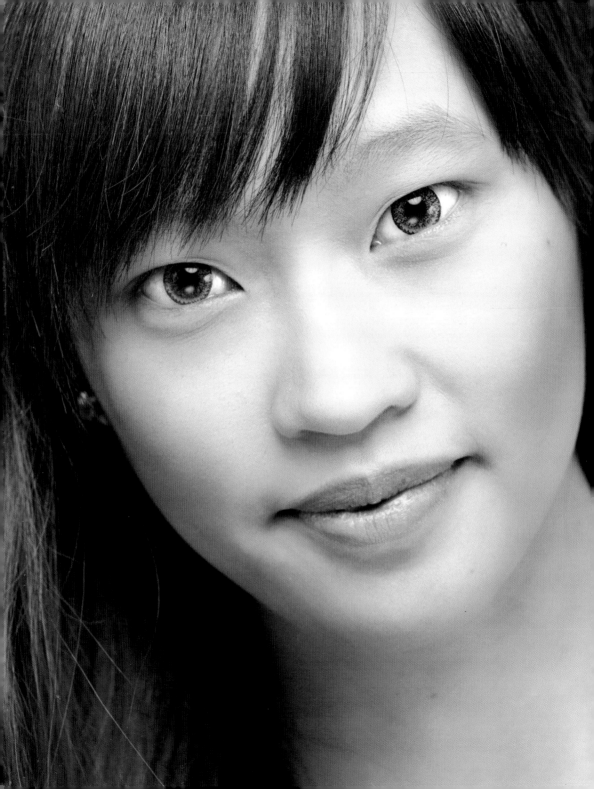

make-up artist, I should know better, even I have suffered the effects of a lazy skincare regime after a long, hard day's work! If I go even one day without my six to eight glasses of water I suffer breakouts, along with dry – and sometimes oily – skin, as my sebaceous glands work overtime trying to rehydrate it.

Lack of sleep, not enough relaxation or exercise are all contributing factors to this problem. It's simple really: live well, feel good and look good!

Prep, prime & moisturise

It is very important to prepare your skin for make-up.

Our skin changes from day to day; hormones, weather and diet all play a part in this. More often than not, I suffer from either oily or combination skin; oily throughout my T-zone (forehead and chin) but dry around my nose.

For years I experimented with different products – and simply everything seemed to bring me out in spots. During one particularly busy week with lots of late nights I removed my make-up with face wipes and cleansed my skin in the morning. My skin actually began to improve. I experimented by using a cleanser at night followed by moisturiser and then washing my face in the morning with water. The change in my routine completely rebalanced my skin!

I realised that what I had been doing was over-cleansing my skin. This had sensitised it, dried it out and caused my oil-producing glands to work overtime to hydrate it. Have you ever noticed that if we wash our hair every day it becomes greasy much more quickly? The same rule applies to our skin.

Cleanse your skin at night with a natural, gentle cleanser, and once in the morning with water. Pat dry with a towel; never scrub or rub the skin on your face as it is very

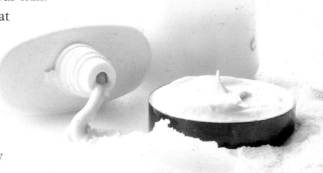

delicate. Again, think of the way we treat our hair. When we go to the hairdresser's they always shampoo our hair twice. The first shampoo rinses away the dirt from the surface of the hair, the second shampoo deep-cleanses the entire head. After shampooing we condition our hair, and now and again we apply a masque for a deep-cleansing treatment. We should apply the same techniques to our skin.

Once a week, remember to exfoliate. This will remove all of the dead skin cells that make our complexion look dull and tired, and reveal the glowing skin beneath. Dry skin is never a good look!

If you have blackheads that you are trying to remove through exfoliation, don't scrub at them – this will actually make them worse. Instead use gentle, circular movements all over your face and neck, avoiding the sensitive eye area, which is very thin and must not be dragged because it can be easily damaged.

Use a face masque once a week to draw out impurities. You can buy masques which deep-cleanse, nourish and hydrate, balance oiliness and brighten tired skin. Once you have determined your skin type you can find a masque which best suits you.

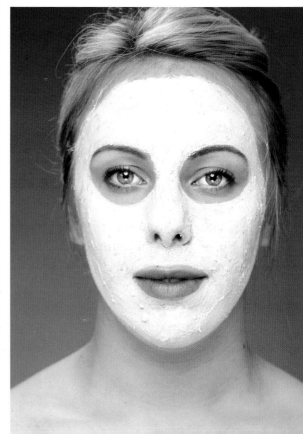

If you wish, pat toner onto your skin using a cotton wool pad. If you don't suffer from oily skin then you don't really need to use this. Always avoid alcohol-based toners as they strip the skin of its natural oils and make it very dry.

Moisturise day and night! Our skin is most active at night, so using a hydrating moisturiser will work wonders. In the morning use a lightweight moisturiser, unless your skin is oily, in which case you can skip moisturiser in the morning and just use it at night. A specific moisturiser may be needed if you have an extremely dry skin or a particular skin condition.

Massage moisturiser into your face and neck using circular, upward motions. Use an eye cream over your delicate eye area. The skin beneath our eyes is very thin, and sometimes is unable to soak in all of the moisture from a facial moisturiser. This can cause puffiness beneath our eyes.

If you suffer from breakouts, acne, pigmentation, redness of the skin or other skin conditions there are products available to target these conditions specifically. I recommend seeing a dermatologist, or your doctor, who can refer you to your nearest skincare specialist.

No matter what your skin type, always use a sunscreen with a high sun protection factor (SPF). Nowadays you can buy face moisturisers and foundations that include an SPF, so you can either apply one of these moisturisers before you put on your make-up, or use a foundation that includes an SPF. SPF foundations are fantastic for helping to prevent sun damage. Combine this with an SPF moisturiser even when the sun is not shining; our skin is still being subjected to harmful ultraviolet (UV) rays which can damage it and potentially cause long-term problems.

Finally, prime your skin before applying foundation. A primer is a silky smooth face serum that creates an even base on which the foundation can sit, while still allowing your skin to breathe.

Understand your own skin

Skin types

After cleansing your skin, and before applying moisturiser, take a close look in the mirror. Is your skin normal, oily, dry, or sensitive? You should assess your skin regularly, as there are many factors, particularly the environment and the weather, that can alter its characteristics. Dry skin, for example, may become oily.

Normal skin: Most commonly seen in young children and babies. The texture is smooth, blemish free and even in colour; pores are very small.

To keep normal skin looking its best, develop the following routine.

- Drink six to eight glasses of water a day.
- Exfoliate once a week.
- Cleanse your skin every morning and night.
- Apply a lightweight moisturiser in the morning.
- Apply a nourishing moisturiser at night.
- Use a lightweight, buildable foundation.
- Eat well and try to get at least eight hours' sleep a night for real benefit.
- Exercise to keep your body happy and healthy.

Oily skin: The skin appears shiny, most obviously through the T-zone (forehead, nose and chin); cheeks may also be oily. This is caused by overactive oil-producing glands. Skin may become increasingly oily towards midday. Pores may look enlarged and excess oil may lead to frequent breakouts, blackheads and/or acne.

Control oily skin with the following routine.

- Drink six to eight glasses of water a day.
- Exfoliate twice a week to minimise the development of blackheads. Do this gently; don't scrub at any blackheads as this may cause more harm than good to the skin.
- Don't over-cleanse your skin; if it becomes too dry it will produce more oil to combat the dryness. Use an oil-free or oil-balancing cleanser at night and then just water in the morning.
- Apply a lightweight, oil-free moisturiser in the morning. Alternatively, if your skin is very oily, you can omit this and use it just at night.
- At night, apply a nourishing but oil-free moisturiser.
- Prep your skin after moisturiser with an oil-free primer.
- Use a lightweight, oil-free foundation, followed by powder to set the product in place. Mineral powders are also great for soaking up excess oil.
- Fixing sprays are brilliant for prolonging the wear of make-up. Spritz it gently

over your face before applying moisturiser. Avoid tinted moisturisers and creamy products – these will just slip straight off your face and appear very shiny.

- Carry blotting papers in your handbag to freshen up throughout the day.
- Eat well and try to get at least eight hours' sleep a night for real benefit.
- Exercise to keep your body happy and healthy.

Dry skin: The skin may appear dull, not radiant. It will appear dry and, in extreme cases, flaky. Texture feels rough to the touch and sometimes bumpy. Skin will feel very tight, especially after cleansing, and the pores are almost invisible. Nourish dry skin with the following routine.

- Drink eight glasses of water a day and eat at least five portions of fruit and vegetables a day to keep the body hydrated.
- Exfoliate twice a week to remove dead skin cells.
- Cleanse skin every morning and night with a gentle, moisturising cleanser.
- Apply a hydrating moisturiser in the morning.
- At night, apply a rich, nourishing moisturiser.
- Try using a foundation balm. This is very much like a tinted moisturiser, with buildable coverage but much more intensive moisture.
- Eat well and try to get at least eight hours' sleep a night for real benefit.
- Exercise to keep your body happy and healthy.

Combination skin: A mixture of dry and oily skin, often oily through the T-zone and dry on the cheeks. Use a mild cleanser and a hydrating moisturiser on dry patches, and an oil-balancing cleanser and lightweight moisturiser on oily areas.

Sensitive skin: Skin is prone to redness, can appear blotchy, and may also itch. Pores may look enlarged. Skin may be susceptible to allergic reactions to cosmetic products. If this is the case, ask your doctor to refer you to a dermatologist, who will be able to offer you advice about specialised products.

Green-based serum may help to reduce the appearance of redness. Use gentle, non-alcohol cleansers, toners and moisturisers. Avoid perfumed products as these can be a major trigger of skin irritation.

Sensitised skin: Can often be confused with sensitive skin. Skin may suffer a brief period of redness caused by a reaction to a particular product; this does not necessarily mean that you have sensitive skin. Use a non-perfumed, natural, lightweight foundation.

Have fun in the sun

When I was at school, all the girls were crazy about getting a tan; at the first glimpse of the English sun we'd be out on the school field, a line of pale legs soaking up the rays. In the summer we'd slip into our bikinis, smother ourselves in baby oil, squeeze lemon juice onto our hair to bleach it under the sun, lay our towels down on the grass and bake for hours. If I burned I used to think, 'Cool, that will look brown tomorrow!' Little did I understand at the time that the sun was actually frying my skin.

Our skin is made up of different layers, and the outer layer – the epidermis – is composed of dead skin cells that are shed about every two weeks. This is why our tans fade over time, as the skin renews itself. It is also the reason why people peel when they tan too quickly.

As for applying lemon juice to my hair – that's just as bad as bathing it in bleach! The citric acid in the fruit strips hair of its natural oils, making it dry and brittle.

It's wonderful to be outside in the warm summer sunshine, as long as we take care not to overdo it. In fact, we need sunshine, as it enables the body to manufacture vitamin D, which is essential for good health. Ideally, we should all see daylight for at least 20 minutes a day, making a special effort throughout the winter months when the days are shorter. Sunshine also stimulates the production of endorphins, which are 'feelgood' chemicals, in our brains – another reason why we feel happier and more optimistic in the summer.

However, the sun's UVA and UVB rays are extremely strong, even when the day may seem cloudy and overcast. These are the rays that cause your tan; they can also cause skin cancer. So, enjoy the sun but take care to protect your skin.

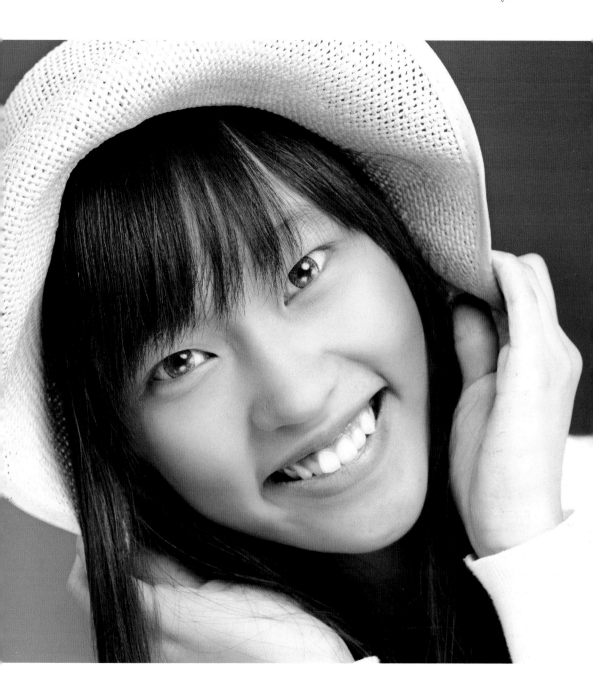

Be bronzed – not burnt!

There is a popular myth that wearing sun lotion stops us from tanning. This is untrue; sun lotion prevents our skin from burning too quickly, allowing us to develop a gradual, long-lasting tan over time. It's a bit like the difference between cooking on a barbecue and cooking in an oven. When we cook food on a barbecue, the heat is so intense that often the food is cooked on the outside before the inside has even had a chance. If we cook food in an oven, gradually it turns evenly golden over a period of time.

During the summer months you should wear a sun lotion with an SPF of at least 15. If you are directly in the sun, reapply it every 20 minutes. Don't forget, if you are swimming in the sea you will burn much more quickly because the light reflects off the water. Check the instructions on your sun lotion to make sure that it is waterproof and how often the manufacturers recommend that you should reapply it.

If you are travelling abroad to a very hot climate take a high-quality sun lotion with you. My sister once travelled to the Dominican Republic where the temperature hit 40 degrees Celsius each day. On her first day there she covered herself in Factor 50, but unfortunately it was a cheap brand and didn't give her enough protection. At the end of the day she began to notice how much her skin was hurting. When we suffer from sunburn our skin continues to react for up to 12 hours. My sister woke up the following morning to find her skin blistered and so painful that she had to seek medical attention. She was left with scars and was unable to leave her hotel room for a week. If you opt for a cheaper brand of sun lotion, take the highest factor you can and apply it frequently.

If your foundation or tinted moisturiser doesn't contain an SPF, remember to buy a moisturiser that does and apply that to your face in the morning. You can also buy SPF lip balms. We often forget about our lips, but they burn too; in fact, the skin on the lips is so thin that they are probably likely to burn first.

Fake tans are the safe option to sunbeds

Once upon a time sunbeds were all the rage. However, this was before people knew so much about the risks and causes of cancer. Today, sensible people choose the safe option of fake tan lotion. These are so much improved that, if they are applied correctly, it can be hard to tell if a tan is real or fake! And not only are they nourishing to your skin, you will avoid the leathery look that comes with too much sun exposure. With fake tan you have the power to look like a bronzed goddess, and stay safe. Follow the tips below and you'll have no white bits, no strap marks, no peeling – just a beautiful, golden glow!

10 steps to the perfect fake tan

1. Exfoliate and moisturise your skin the day before your tan to remove all of your dead skin cells. Pay special attention to your elbows, knees and ankles as these tend to be dry areas. Use a gentle face exfoliant on your face; the particles in body scrubs are far too rough.

2. Shave or wax at least 24 hours before your tan. This enables your skin to settle down and prevents infection in open pores.

3. Remove all of your make-up, deodorant and perfume before tanning as they can create a barrier between your skin and the tanning lotion.

4. Use a mitt with all fake tanning lotions (unless you are having a spray tan done professionally) as it gives an even distribution of colour and a streak-free tan.

5. Begin by applying fake tan to your legs, and work up your body, finishing with your face. This will prevent you smudging, streaking or accidentally removing any of the tan you have already applied.

6. Before you tan your hands or feet, apply moisturiser or barrier cream to your palms and

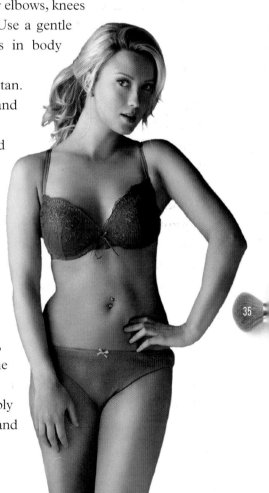

the soles of your feet, and in between your fingers and toes, to avoid tanning them.

7. Allow the tan to dry and then wear loose, dark clothing immediately after you have finished, to avoid the tan rubbing off onto light-coloured clothes..

8. Avoid wearing any tight footwear, socks or underwear that may rub the tan off.

9. Leave the tan on for a minimum of six to eight hours before washing and wait two to three hours before washing your hands. If any part of you does get wet, pat – don't rub – it dry.

10. Once your tan is set, and you have showered, moisturise your skin every day to prolong your tan for as long as possible.

Remember that most fake tan lotions do not contain an SPF, so you still need to protect your skin in the sun.

How to choose your make-up

It is natural to be tempted by cheap make-up but, remember, it is cheap for a reason and not always good value. Expensive products are generally very long-lasting on your skin so, although you pay more, the bottle will last for at least the same amount of time, if not longer than a cheaper, lower-quality make-up that has to be reapplied often.

When choosing your make-up, check the ingredients as some brands are packed full of chemicals, many of which may not be good for your skin. In particular, try to avoid buying any products containing parabens as there is some evidence that these could be harmful.

If you are on a tight budget, don't forget that classy make-up makes a great present. So, next time someone asks you what you would like for a gift, grab the chance to choose a fabulous product you wouldn't be able to afford to buy yourself.

Learn how to apply make-up properly. Lessons are always available with make-up artists, or you can pop to any of your local department store make-up counters and arrange a free makeover. You will gain expert advice on what is available, what suits you, why you should use particular products and how to apply them.

Experiment to discover what you like and what suits you.

How often should you replace your make-up?

Just like any other product, make-up has a shelf life. It's really important to take note of 'use by' dates because out-of-date products can cause your skin to become irritated. Over time, too, they become less effective and don't wear so well.

The following list is a guide to the average life of the most popular products.

Mascara	3–6 months
Eye pencils	12–18 months
Eyeshadow	2 years
Eye cream	6 months
Liquid and cream foundation	2 years
Concealer	2 years
Powder	2 years
Powder blusher	2 years
Cream blusher	2 years
Lipstick	12–18 months
Sunscreen	2 years
Face cream	2 years

Assessing your skin tone

Skin tones vary considerably from person to person, but most people fall into one of the following groups.

Fair skin: Very light, generally does not tan quickly, if at all; prone to sunburn. Some people have lots of freckles. Generally suits alabaster or porcelain shades of foundation (the lightest colours).

Olive skin: Darker in colour and tans easily.

Dark skin: Ranges from light brown to black.

Is your skin cool or warm?

Identifying the undertone colour of your skin is an important part of colour matching make-up for your skin.

The best way to identify the undertone of your skin is by looking at your natural hair colour. If your hair colour is warm (hints of golden, bronze or copper), your skin undertone is warm.

If your hair colour is ashy, with no golden, bronze or copper shades, then your undertone is cool.

Warm skin tends to look more golden and peachy, while fair skin tends to look more ashy and pale.

Choosing the right make-up colours

☐ I honestly believe that any colour can suit anyone if they choose the right shade.
☐ If you have cool, fair skin, choose pastel colours.
☐ If you have warm, darker skin you can choose warmer, brighter or darker colours.

> **Tip:** Silvers can be made to look warm – mix with a hint of gold or warm brown.

Cool colours   **Warm colours**

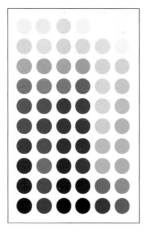
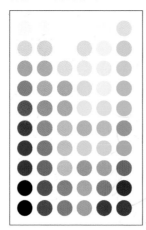

38

CHAPTER 3

The Perfect Base

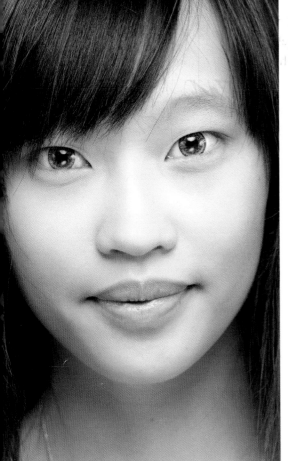

Primer formulas

Before an artist begins to paint, they prep their canvas with a formula specific to what they are creating. This ensures a smooth, even base for them to work on. A primer does the same thing for your skin. It evens out skin tone, minimises pores and blemishes, balances the oils in your skin and creates a long-lasting, smooth base for your foundation to sit on. It contains properties that soak up excess oils, so that your foundation will stay on for longer. I also believe that, while still allowing your skin to breathe, a primer helps it by creating a barrier between skin and foundation. This means that, rather than soaking into your pores, the foundation will sit nicely on the surface of your skin, creating a healthier base for you.

Primers are available in cream and serum formulas. Creams are thicker and are better for dry skin that needs some additional hydration, although personally I find them a little too thick on oily skin.

Serums are fabulous for oily skin, as they are lightweight and generally oil free. You can also purchase specific oil-free primers which have an extra boost. Even if you decide not to wear foundation and you just want to stick to your bronzer and blusher, make sure you use your primer first so that the powder will stay put. If you brush powder products onto bare skin it will brush straight off again.

Foundation formulas

There are so many different foundation formulas available that sometimes the choice can be a bit overwhelming. They cater for every skin type, whether normal,

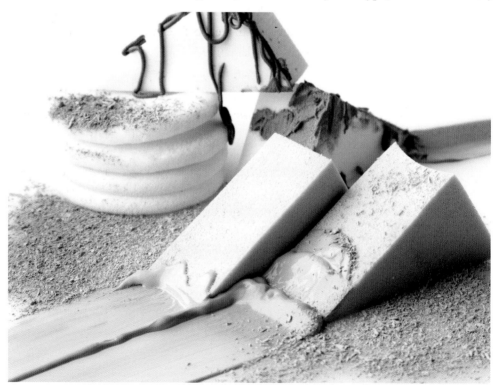

dry, combination or oily. Below are descriptions of the various formulas that you can buy, to help you identify more clearly which type will best suit your skin type.

Coverage

- **Full** – Gives a flawless finish. Covers most scars, blemishes and pigmentation. Great for dark skin tones. The product can be mixed with a moisturiser to make it sheerer.

- **Medium** – My personal favourite. Less thick in consistency but can be built to give full coverage without looking cakey. Lets your natural skin tone shine through.

- **Sheer** – Emphasises your natural skin tone. A translucent coverage which still evens skin tone. Gives a beautiful make-up-free effect that's fantastic on holiday if you don't want to go bare-faced!

Formulas

- **Tinted moisturiser** – Provides a completely natural look, great for normal and dry skin types.

- **Tinted face balm** – Nourishes extremely dry skin, giving a natural, dewy look.

- **Foundation stick** – Gives great coverage, brilliant for covering blemishes and evening out skin tone. Can be a little greasy for oily skin, which may cause the product to slip. Fabulous for all other skin types.

- **Liquid foundation** – These are brilliant for all skin types. Liquid-to-powder or oil-free formulas are perfect for oily skin; illuminating or hydrating formulas give dry skin a radiant glow. They are available in light, medium and full coverage consistencies.

◻ **Cream foundation** – Medium to full coverage, available in both hydrating and oil-free formulas. Perfect for nourishing dry skin.

◻ **Mineral foundation** – Brilliant for soaking up excess oil. I adore using mineral products over liquid foundation as a concealer. Check the ingredients are natural. Avoid any talc-based products; talc is very ageing over time because it dries your skin out so much.

◻ **Mousse** – A whipped foundation that gives a matt finish. Although this product feels light on your skin, I find it gives quite heavy coverage. Use only a little at a time, as its light but thick consistency makes it more prone to caking onto your skin.

Highlighter formulas

Highlighters are used to enhance your features and face. There are three main formulas available to buy:

◻ **Liquid** – Great for emphasising dewy skin.

◻ **Cream** – Great for emphasising dewy skin, supereasy to blend. Use on eyes too for a gorgeous sheen!

◻ **Powder** – Works perfectly on matt skin (skin with no shine).

I find the best way to apply highlighter is to use your fingers. You have direct control over what you are doing, and the warmth of your fingers helps to blend the product into your skin.

The secret to perfect highlighter

I have discovered that the secret to perfect highlighter is to apply it *beneath* your foundation. This gives your skin a glow without making you look artificial. If you find the effect isn't dewy enough you can apply more once your make-up is complete.

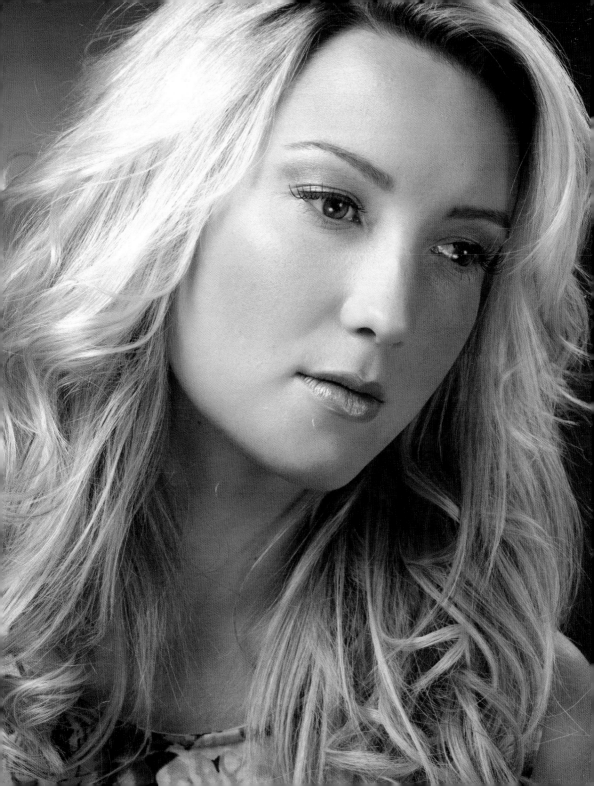

Powder formulas

Powder is used to remove unwanted shine and give your skin a matt look. It also sets your make-up to give it longer-lasting wear.

Powder is available in two different forms:

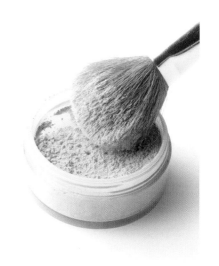

Compact: This comes as a block of powder, and is great if you only want a light dusting.

Loose powder: Loose powder is brilliant for creating a matt look, and for getting rid of excess oil.

Whichever formula you prefer, both are available either in different shades or as translucent powder. I would always opt for translucent because it is colourless.

Tools for applying foundation

As with any other precise, detailed work, it's important to have the correct tools for applying and blending your make-up.

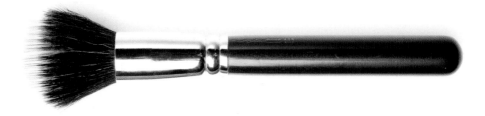

44

Multi-use brush: My favourite for applying foundation. Its full, fluffy bristles allow you to apply your foundation in a circular motion giving light weight.

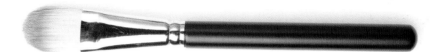

Foundation brush: This is a full, flat-edged brush with synthetic bristles. It distributes foundation evenly and allows you to layer the product.

Sponges: Disposable wedge-shaped sponges are the best. The corners allow you to cover hard-to-reach areas like the corners of the nose. They are fantastic for applying foundation thoroughly and for blending it seamlessly. Also great for applying concealer.

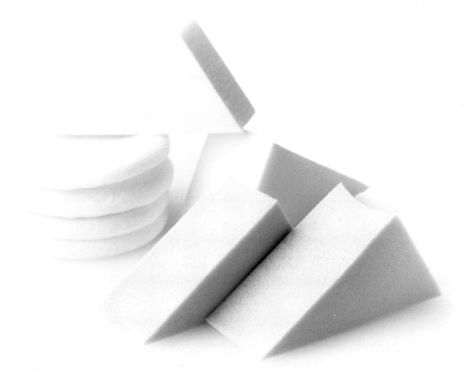

Fingers: Your fingers allow you direct control of the product and the warmth of your hands warms the product, allowing it to glide easily onto the skin. Be sure to cleanse your hands and nails before doing this.

Use a **big fluffy brush** to apply your bronzer and blusher. The brush head should be large enough to cover the apple of your cheek.

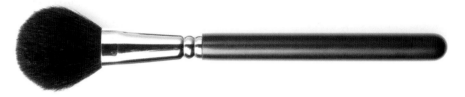

Very important: You must always remember to clean your brushes after you use them – every time. This helps to prevent the spread of bacteria which can cause infections and spots on your skin. Imagine wiping a brush over spots day after day . . .

If you share brushes with your friends, remember to clean them after each person has used them. You can buy brush cleansing spray at any of the department store make-up counters. Just spritz a little onto a cotton pad and swirl it over your brush until it is clean.

Once every couple of weeks give your brushes a thorough cleanse with brush shampoo. Again you can buy this from any department store make-up counter. Try not to leave the brushes soaking in warm water as this tends to soften the glue and inevitably the brush heads will fall apart.

Where possible, I think young girls should avoid foundation, although I understand that lack of confidence encourages us to want to cover up flaws and blemishes. With my step- by-step guide to perfect application, you will learn to create a flawless-looking complexion without plastering on the make-up.

How does foundation work?

As I have explained, foundation is used to even out skin tone. It does this by minimising areas of redness on your skin, as well as blemishes and spots. Never try to cover freckles though! Freckles are beautiful and trying to cover them can result in skin that looks chalky.

In my experience there is never any need for thick foundation; it just looks cakey and mask-like on your skin. Instead opt for a more natural, lightweight formula. The secret to evening out your skin is in layering the product and building it up gradually. It's much like painting your nails: the first coat can look wishy-washy, while the second will be much deeper and cover the nail completely. Remember that the most beautiful skin is natural-looking skin.

You don't need to use foundation all over your face unless your skin tone is particularly uneven. Only use it on areas that need it. If your skin tone is nice and even, don't use it at all; allow your skin to breathe and be beautiful.

If you suffer from acne don't try to cover up spots with heavy make-up as this looks very unnatural and will actually draw attention to them. I'll show you the technique for disguising spots later in this chapter.

Very important: Foundation is not designed to make your face look tanned! *Always* use a foundation that matches your skin tone exactly. If you don't you will end up with tide lines around the bottom of your jaw, and will look as if you are wearing a mask. Orange foundation is never flattering.

Instead choose a foundation with yellow, rather than pink, undertones. This is because most people have yellow undertones in their skin, so a yellow-based foundation will look most natural. The yellow also helps to hide any redness in the skin because yellow and red are complementary colours which help to balance each other out. Pink undertones tend to look very obvious on the skin.

There are a few people, such as redheads, whose very fair skin may have pink undertones, but I find that using an alabaster or porcelain shade works perfectly for them, as it hides any pink that needs to be toned down. If you are unsure about choosing a shade to suit your own skin, seek advice from a professional or department store make-up artist.

Bronzer is used to give you a 'sun-kissed' bronze goddess look. Avoid using bronzer if you have cool, porcelain skin, as it tends to look muddy. Instead opt for a peach or light pink shade of blusher to give you a healthy, natural glow. If you want to contour your face, use a slightly darker shade of foundation in these areas.

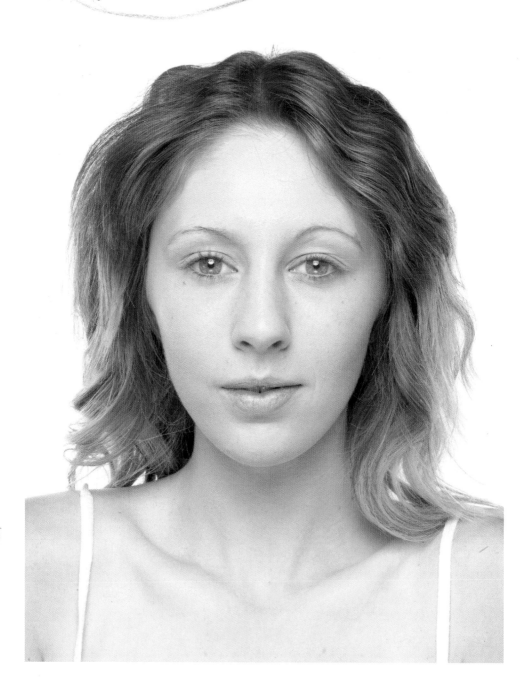

How to apply your foundation perfectly

Blend, blend, blend – there must never be any visible lines showing when you have applied your foundation! No tide lines, please, girls; if your colour is correct and you have blended the product seamlessly into your skin, you should see no colour marks at all.

Always prep your skin with a foundation primer, to smooth and even it out and to help make your foundation last longer.

Look at your skin in the mirror; what areas need covering?

Test your foundation shade along your jawline and slightly down onto your neck; the shade should match both. Often the skin on our face is darker than that on our neck, because our face tends to cast a shadow over our neck and shield it from the sun. If this is the case, use one shade for your face, and a lighter one to hide any lines on your neck, and blend the two until you can't see any difference. If you own a lighter foundation and a slightly darker one you can mix the two to create your perfect shade. If you do this, test the colour on your chest, as the skin here is commonly the same colour as on the face, especially in the summer.

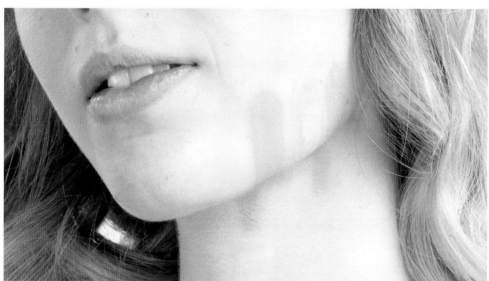

Small areas

If you only need to cover small areas of your face, use a small amount of foundation at a time and pat it on the area that you want to even out. Build up the coverage in layers until you are happy with the way it looks. You can also use a foundation brush or sponge if you prefer.

The whole face

If you prefer to use foundation over your entire face, begin with a small amount. Using either your fingers, a brush or a sponge, blend it from your hairline, down your forehead, down onto your nose, onto your cheeks and then down towards your chin. Blend the colour right down onto your neck until it is invisible. You must not be able to see any lines!

Once you have applied your first layer, you can build up layers in the areas where you need more coverage until you are happy with the result. If you layer it well you may be able to hide spots with foundation alone; if not, use a concealer or a foundation stick, which is thicker than normal foundation, on the areas that need it.

Tip: If you want an even more natural look, try mixing your foundation with a little of your daytime moisturiser and apply it like a tinted moisturiser. This technique evens out your skin tone without any foundation being visible on the surface of your skin. It really does work!

What is the difference between concealer and corrector?

Concealers cover up flaws and blemishes you don't want people to notice; correctors lighten and brighten. They are a thin, creamy consistency, perfect for under the eyes. You need to set both with translucent powder between applications.

Conceal your spots

If you suffer from spots and blemishes, don't panic; there are tricks you can use to hide them.

Choose a shade of concealer that matches your skin colour perfectly; make sure that it is no lighter as this will only make the blemish more obvious. Use a synthetic brush, or a clean finger, and dot the product onto the area or spot that you want to cover. Wipe away or blend any extra product surrounding the blemish and then fix the concealer into place with a dusting of translucent powder. Translucent power is uncoloured, so it won't alter the colour of your skin.

If you have bad acne, and don't want to leave it uncovered, use exactly the same technique but keep building up the concealer until you can no longer see the blemish.

I would recommend using a special medicinal concealer, such as those available from the Dermacolor range by Kryolan. These will help the skin to heal while also giving good coverage. The chemicals in standard concealers may make your skin break out further.

For even greater camouflage, you can also use a mineral foundation dotted over the concealer. The combination of the concealer's creamy consistency and the foundation's powder gives really great, lasting coverage. The minerals in the foundation are medicinal and so treat the spot at the same time.

If you have darkness under your eyes don't use thick spot concealer to cover it. The skin under your eyes is thinner and lighter than the rest of your skin, so you need to use a light-reflective corrector and pat it into the dark areas, from the inner to the outer corner of each eye.

What colour correctors do I need?
As a professional make-up artist, I find that skin correctors and perfecters are a vital part of my kit.

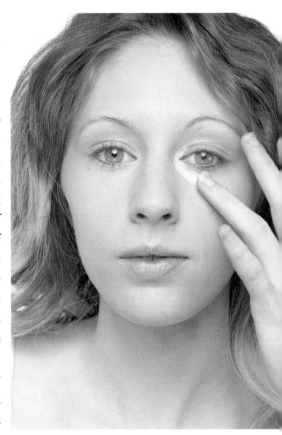

I tend to stick to three main colours – green, yellow and orange. Think back to art classes at school when you learned about complementary colours: green neutralises red, so this is the colour that you will use to reduce the appearance of reddened spots, blemishes and areas of skin. I find it particularly great on acne rosacea. Dermologica do a fabulous one called Sheer Tint Redness Relief which is not only SPF15 but also contains medicinal ingredients to help to relieve the problem.

Yellow/peach neutralises the blue/grey appearance beneath our eyes. The skin is very thin and translucent here in comparison to the rest of the face, so our veins create a blue/grey/green tinge beneath our eyes. The trick is to make the skin look more opaque.

Orange is brilliant for neutralising any brown pigmentation or extremely dark areas under the eyes, especially on Asian or black skin tones.

How do I use correctors?

Here are a few top tricks of the trade for using your perfecter and concealer.

Start by analysing your skin in the mirror. Remember, you are not looking to mask your skin, you want your natural beauty to glow through. All you are trying to do is create an even skin tone to project a flawless effect. No one has completely blemish-free skin, so don't try to hide moles or other characteristics that make you unique. Once you have decided what needs to be improved, choose the appropriate colour corrector.

An under eye perfecter lightens and brightens the face to give it a healthy glow. So, if you have barely any darkness, use one shade lighter than your natural skin tone to give it a really fresh appearance. Use your ring finger to pat a small amount from the inner corner of your eye down beneath your lower lashes, covering the translucent area.

If you suffer from tired-looking eyes use the same technique but first pat a yellow perfecter into the dark areas. You only need a small amount of this; you don't want to look like a character from *The Simpsons*! Blend the colour back to your natural tone by adding a skin-coloured perfecter over the top. Finish with a skin-brightening powder such as Laura Mercier's Secret Brightening Powder, which will also set the perfecter and prevent it from creasing.

Finally, if you suffer from very dark under eyes, or black/brown pigmentation, use the same technique but with an orange or peach perfecter. You can mix it with yellow to make it lighter, depending on your skin tone. Follow this with a skin-coloured perfecter and your brightening powder.

If you are covering pigmentation or blemishes with a concealer, use your finger, brush or a sponge to pat it lightly over the blemished area. Build up the concealer in layers and pat each layer with translucent powder to fix it in place.

Creating matt skin (skin with no shine)

This look is often popular during the winter months when skin is paler and clothes are darker in colour and heavier in texture.

Dust translucent powder all over your face and build it up until you have the desired effect. A little goes a long way, so don't dust too much on at once or your face will look caked. Use a brush to do this. Tap your brush on the edge of your pot or on the back of your hand to get rid of the excess powder before you sweep it over your face. Start from your hairline and move in towards the centre of your face.

Creating dewy skin (skin with lots of healthy shine)

This look is often popular throughout the summer months when skin is bronzed and shimmering, and clothes are light in colour and texture.

If you want dewy skin with lots of healthy shine, only use powder on the areas where make-up needs setting, such as your T-zone – your forehead, nose and chin – which is often oilier than cheeks. Smile and blend a cream blusher over the apples of your cheeks, along the tops of your cheekbones, stopping at your temples. Make sure it is blended seamlessly, with no visible lines.

Pat a cream highlighter along the very tops of your cheekbones, up over your temples and round to the outer corner of your eyebrows in a C shape.

Alternatively, you can skip the highlighter and instead use an illuminating moisturiser underneath your foundation in the areas that you want to look highlighted.

Learn how to contour your face

What does contouring mean?

Contouring means shading and highlighting an image to make it look three-dimensional. For example, if you draw a portrait of someone, you use shading and highlighting to create the face. If you were just to draw outlines, the image would look flat. The same technique is used in make-up, when you shade and highlight your face using bronzer and highlighter.

The first step in learning how to contour is to understand where on your face you need to shade, and where you need to highlight.

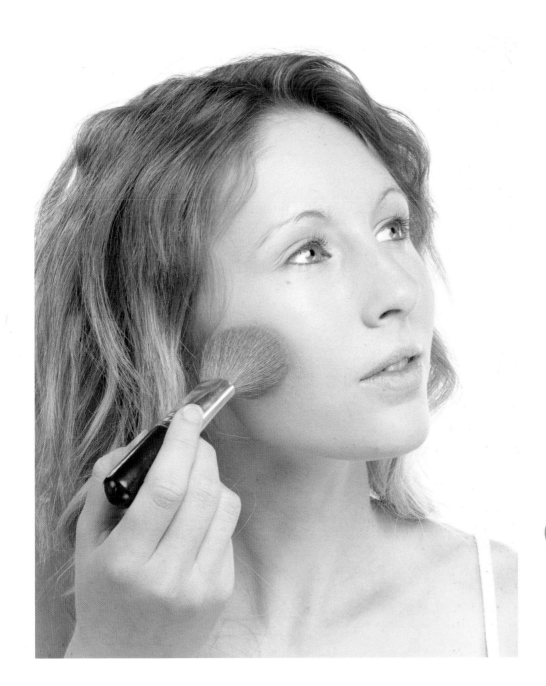

55

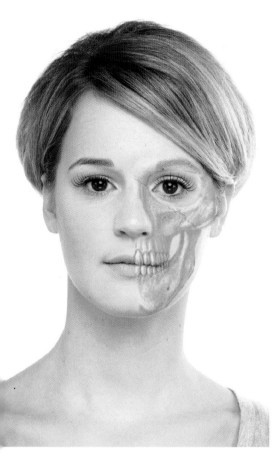

Take a look at the image shown here of the human bone structure. The dark areas that lie beneath the bones are where you would shade your face. The light areas, such as the tops of your cheekbones, you would leave unshaded, or highlight.

Try experimenting with this on your own or someone else's face. Notice how shading and highlighting certain areas can change the way you look.

For example, by shading the end of a long nose you can make it appear shorter; by shading down either side of a wide nose you can make it appear thinner. If you highlight down the centre of your nose you can create the illusion of a straighter, smaller nose. Highlighting the hairline of a small forehead will make it appear larger.

To create the illusion of higher cheekbones, shade the hollows of your cheeks. Suck in your cheeks like a fish and shade the hollowed areas directly beneath your cheekbones.

Highlighting

Highlighter is used on areas that the light would naturally hit, such as the tops of our cheekbones, our foreheads and our noses.

Always begin by mapping out your highlighted areas. It's entirely up to you whether you apply highlighter before or after applying your foundation. The areas that are most usually highlighted are towards the centre of your face: central forehead, brow bones, the centre of your nose bone (stop before the tip of your nose), your chin and the tops of your cheekbones and temples.

Shading

Shading your face correctly will emphasise the highlights. Once you've practised this a few times you will automatically begin to know where you need to highlight, where you need to shade, and whether you're getting it right or wrong.

Suck in your cheeks and study your face. Notice where your skin hollows; these are the areas that you should shade. Sweep your bronzer into the dips in your cheeks, across your hairline, down the sides of your nose, over your chin and down your neck. Take a fluffy brush and blend all of the edges away. You must blend seamlessly to avoid an artificial look. Once this is done, sweep a clean brush over your entire face to ensure that you have left no patches, and then sweep the brush underneath your eyes to make sure that you are not left with white panda eyes.

Take a photo and see what you think.

Contouring different face shapes

- **Full face –** sweep bronzer lightly along your hairline.

- **To emphasise high cheekbones –** sweep blusher over the apples of your cheeks and up towards your temples.

- **Round face –** make a round face look slimmer by shading beneath your cheekbones and a little either side of your chin. Sweep blusher over the apples of your cheeks.

- **Square face –** soften the angles of your face by sweeping bronzer over your forehead, cheekbones, jaw, chin and eyelids.

- **Rectangular face –** apply bronzer to the tops of your cheekbones.

- **Oval face –** sweep blusher over the tops of your cheekbones and softly over the apples of your cheeks.

57

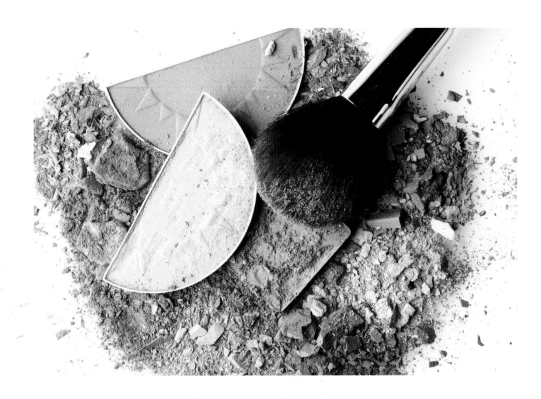

58

Bronzer/blusher formulas

◻ **Compressed powder:** Tidy and easy to blend.

◻ **Loose powder:** Easy to blend, less is more.

◻ **Cream:** Very natural, blends into the skin seamlessly. Can be used on eyes and lips too.

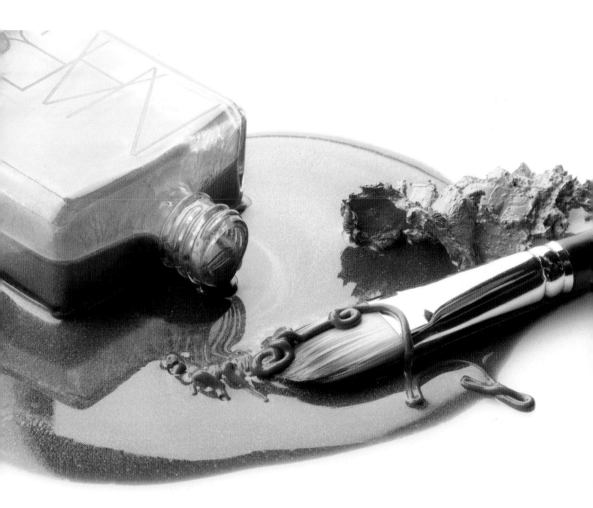

Tint: Can be tricky to use and has to be blended very quickly. Good for shading areas of your face such as underneath your cheekbones to make them look higher.

Gel: Easy to blend, lovely on foundation-free, natural skin.

Applying your bronzer

Bronzer is used to make your skin look healthy and glowing. Use it on all areas of your face that would naturally catch the sun; for example, your forehead, nose, under your cheekbones (not above), on the apples of your cheeks, on your chin and neck. If you are using a powder bronzer, dust your skin with translucent powder first to ensure that the bronzer goes on smoothly. If you try and dust bronzer onto oily skin it will look patchy where the product clings to the oily areas.

Swirl your brush through the bronzer, tap off excess powder and blend it in so that you can't see any lines.

If you are going to use a cream, tint or gel, ensure that you apply it before using any powder on your face. If you try to apply a liquid or gel product over powder it will look caked on and uneven.

If you have very pale skin, opt for a peachy bronzer rather than brown. Pale skin tends not to tan, so a brown bronzer will look fake and muddy. Peach will make your skin glow.

Build bronzer up slowly. If you put too much on in one go it will make your skin look orange, powdery and unnatural.

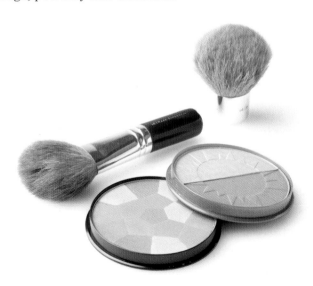

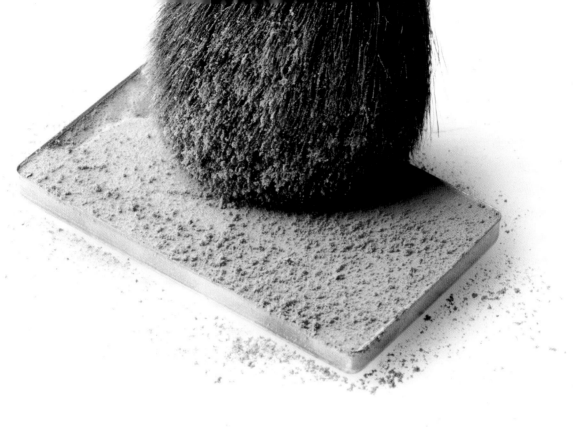

Applying your blusher

Blusher gives you a healthy glow. Try to match the colour that you turn when you exercise, as this will look the most natural.

Using a brush, dust your face with translucent powder and then smile and dust the blusher onto the apples of your cheeks. Blend it up towards your hairline along the top of your cheekbones, but don't go too close to your eyes or nose. Keep the blusher a fingertip space away from them or it will look over the top, unnatural and unflattering.

Cream blusher looks the most natural because you can't see it on the surface of your skin. Cheek stains are also very good. Although these products may take a little time to get perfect, they are applied to exactly the same areas as powder blushers. Instead of using a brush, though, use the warmth of your fingers to blend the product into your skin.

Never use blusher on any part of your face other than your cheekbones. If you try to contour your face with a blusher your make-up will look very dated! Stick to bronzers for this technique.

> Tip: **To** make your blusher last longer, blend a cream blush into your cheeks, sweep a dusting of translucent powder over the top and then a sweep of powder blusher over the top of this. If you want to add more depth to your glow, apply a brighter powder blusher on the apples of your cheeks to make them ping.

Foundation is great for evening out the skin tone, but the effect can be a little flat without bronzer, blusher or highlighter to emphasise cheekbones and add contouring to the face. Remember, we use bronzer or a darker shade of foundation to shade our faces, and highlighter or a lighter shade of foundation to highlight our faces.

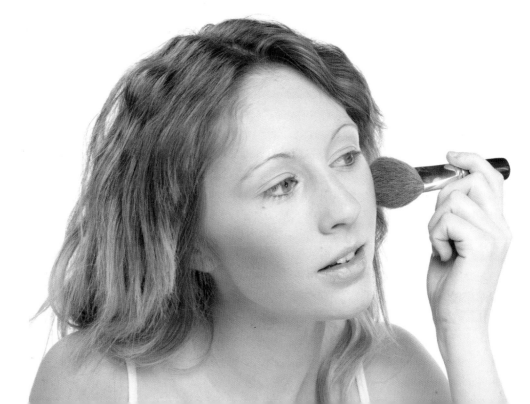

CHAPTER 4

Emphasise your Eyes

Eyeshadow formulas

Eyeshadows have the power to completely change a look. You can turn a very natural make-up into a much bolder one just by the sweep of an eyeshadow. Below are some of the most common types of eyeshadow available.

- **Eye primer:** Ensures that the eyeshadow remains long lasting and crease-free.
- **Gloss:** Creates shine.
- **Cream:** Silky, smooth and easy to apply.
- **Mousse:** A cream-to-powder finish.
- **Compressed powder:** Strong colour and definition, easy to blend.
- **Loose-pigment powder:** Bright colours and easy to blend.
- **Aqua colour:** Mixed with water to create an extreme colour; a lot like face paint.
- **Greasepaint:** Very strong pigment, completely opaque, must be set with powder. Great for fancy dress!

Tools that you can use to apply eye make-up

Eye shader brush: Wide, flat bristles that can sweep shadow from the lash line to the brow bone.

Eyeshadow brush: Natural, soft, rounded bristles, sweeps shadow across the lower lid.

Eye contour brush: Round head with flat bristles made from natural hair. Bristles are short and dense, great for applying shadow to the crease.

Eye blender brush: Soft and fluffy bristles, fantastic for blending shadow.

Eye smudge brush: Small, soft, flexible bristles with a rounded end. Great for smudging eyeliner for a smoky eye look.

Flat eyeliner brush: Flat, synthetic bristles, slightly round head, perfect for shadow liner.

Eyeliner brush, ultra fine: Synthetic bristles curved to a point. Perfect for gel liner application.

Brow brush: Short, stiff bristles cut on an angle. Used for tidying brows and applying shadow to the brows. Make sure that the bristles are a mixture of synthetic and natural. 100% synthetic would be too stiff to hold eyeshadow.

Synthetic bristle brush: Great for applying cream or mousse eyeshadow.

Eyelash comb: used for separating the lashes.

Eyelash curler: Used to curl the lashes before applying mascara or false lashes.

Never use those little sponge applicators you are given in eyeshadow kits; they don't apply the eyeshadow evenly, or blend at all well.

It is said that our eyes are the windows to our souls. When we meet someone that we like, it all starts with a glance, then a gaze into each other's eyes. When we talk to people, eye contact is what creates a connection.

All eye make-up is designed to help you make the most of your eyes. With the right make-up you can create whatever mood and atmosphere you choose.

Before you apply any eyeshadow, ensure that loose shadow does not fall onto your beautifully prepped base by dotting loose powder beneath your eyes, following your lower lash line. This will catch and collect the colour as it falls. Brush the powder away very gently once you have finished applying your eyeshadow.

Natural eye make-up that suits everyone

The basic eye make-up is a style that suits everyone, emphasising shape, colour and beauty. Any colour or shade can be used to create this look, taking into account each individual person's features, eye colour and skin tone.

I have found that whether your skin is fair or dark, and whatever colour your eyes are, neutral tones will always flatter them, which is why you will often see these on brides.

Browns, golds, peaches, warm greys and bronze all flatter any skin tone, provided that the right shade is chosen. The right colour and shade will enhance your skin tone, make your eyes look brighter and lift your face. Avoid red-based shadows though as these can make your eyes look sore.

For a very natural look, sweep a light, natural shade similar to your own skin colour over your eyelid, and then use a slightly darker shade, or a shimmery shade, over your eyelid and into the crease of your eye, and blend. Apply mascara.

For a slightly more sophisticated look, note the basic three-shade rule:

light;
medium;
dark.

First prime your eyes, all over your eyelids and up to your brow bone. You can use your fingers for this or a synthetic bristle brush.

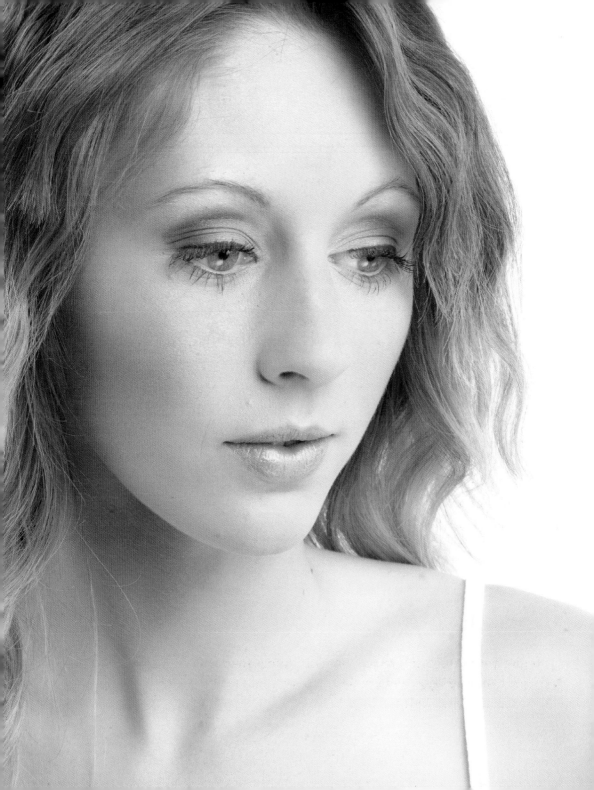

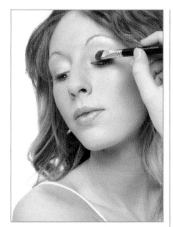
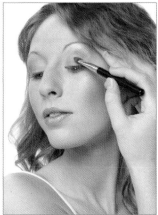
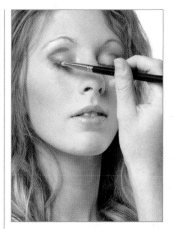

Next, take a light base shade over your eyelids, right up to your brow bone. Use an eyeshadow brush for this. Matt shades are great, too, but can appear a little flat unless brows are highlighted. Pop a small amount of cream highlighter or powder shimmer just beneath your brows on the brow bone.

Sweep your medium shade over your eyelids and into the crease of each eye, using your eyeshadow brush. Blend completely with your eye blender brush.

Using your darkest shade, draw a backwards V shape in the outer corner of each eye with your eye contour brush, as shown in the picture. Blend, following your natural crease line, with your eye blender brush. Be sure not to take the eyeshadow further than the outer corner of each eye, otherwise this can have the effect of dragging your eyes down.

To give your eyes even greater emphasis, take a fourth shade, which should be deeper than your dark shade, and blend it only into the very outer corner of your lower lid in another little V shape.

When you apply shadow, pat the product onto your eyelids with your brush before you blend; this gives an even distribution of colour and allows it to sit on the skin without looking wishy-washy.

If you are using cream shadows, stick solely to cream, metallic or shimmery shadows throughout the application. Mixing cream shadow with matt powder shadow can result in a caked and unnatural look.

Leave your bottom lashes free from mascara and smudge a small amount of dark shadow into the outer corner of each eye.

Pay attention to eyebrows and always keep them tidy. Use a shadow the same colour as your natural eyebrows to fill them in; powder looks soft and natural. You can buy fantastic brow set sticks (they look a lot like mascara tubes but contain a clear gel) to keep any wild hairs in place!

Asian eyes

If you have Asian eyes without a crease, don't try to draw one in. You can create the illusion of depth by sweeping a light shadow over your lid, using a medium one in the inner corners of your eyes, and a dark shade on the outer corners. Sweep outwards horizontally to create shadow.

Asian eyes are beautiful as they are; defining the shape of the lower lid is what looks most natural.

If you are Asian and have large, beautiful eyes with a crease you can be as

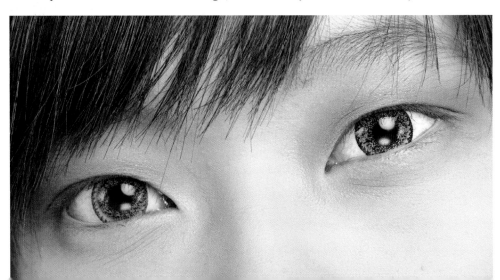

creative as you like with colour and shape. Your eyes often look their most beautiful when they are really emphasised. Try defining the crease with some bold shadowing!

If you wear glasses

Don't feel as if you have to pile on make-up behind your glasses to draw attention to your eyes. Glasses have now become such a fashion item that they add instant glamour to your looks. All you need to do is define your eyes, so keep your brows tidy and apply your eyeshadow in the usual way, but just enhance the colour slightly more than is usual. If you opt for natural-looking eyes, try teaming them with bright lips for a superfunky look.

Eyeliner

Eyeliner is brilliant for making our eyes stand out, and you can apply it in several different ways to create a variety of effects.

A trick I love is to use two colours: for example, purple along your top lash line and turquoise along the bottom. Try making a statement using your favourite colours. If you want to take it even further, add a coloured mascara to your lashes.

Lower your eyelid, gently hold the skin taut and apply eyeliner right into your lash line. Using small strokes, begin in the middle and sweep to the outer edge of your eye. Finish the line by sweeping from the innermost corner of your eye to join the line you started in the middle.

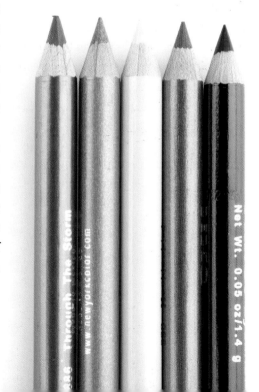

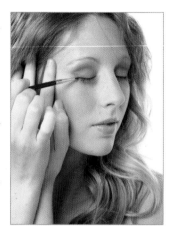

☐ Liner shadow mixed with eyeliner sealer creates a natural but flattering emphasis on your eyes.

☐ Gel liner creates a bold or dramatic eye.

☐ Pencil liner and dry shadow are great for lining your lower lashes, especially for a smoky eye effect.

☐ To make your eyes appear brighter, apply liner only on the top lashes for a fresh look.

☐ Lining the inside rim of your eyes with dark liner makes them appear smaller.

☐ Lining the inside rim of your eyes with white liner makes them appear larger.

I wouldn't recommend lining the inner rim of your eyes unless you are trying to create a very dramatic effect, or wish to make very large eyes appear smaller, as it can be dangerous. If you want to line your lower lashes on the outer edge, use a kohl pencil and smudge it across. Using a liquid eyeliner looks far too dark and hard and makes the inner rims of your eyes appear red and sore. If you are adamant that you do want to use liquid along the bottom you must line the inner rim of your eyes with a dark or light pencil to balance your eyes and keep them looking sparkly. Be very gentle when you apply this. If you do line the inner rim, use a kohl liner, as these are generally manufactured with antibacterial qualities and will have been tested. Never line the inner rim with liquid or gel – this will sting and can be dangerous!

    If you want a completely natural look but still want your eyes to look defined, try using a thin, flat eyeliner brush. Place the brush right at the roots of your upper lashes and wiggle the brush through them. This technique will line between your lashes rather than create a hard line on your eyelid. If you do decide to apply eyeliner as a thin line, you can use a dry brush to soften the line afterwards and smudge it out ever so slightly.

There are lots of ways you can play around with your eyeliner: use different colours; change the shape of your eyes – for instance, create cat's eyes by flicking up the outer corners; make it thicker for more drama.

Mascara

Girls always ask me, 'What is the best mascara?'

The truth is that everyone has a different opinion. Mascaras that lengthen and volumise are most popular; however, it all depends on what works for you and what look you are trying to achieve. In my experience, an expensive mascara is not necessarily better than one made by a cheaper brand.

I love high-volume and definition mascara that gives sleek and smooth results. It shapes and defines to create long, beautiful lashes, and you get perfect separation with no clumping. Define your look, naturally!

Always read the label on your mascara to make sure it is suitable for sensitive eyes and wearers of contact lenses. Some mascaras contain fibres which can irritate your eyes.

Very important: Never share mascara, as this can spread bacteria which cause eye infections such as conjunctivitis. If you want to share you can buy disposable mascara wands which can be thrown away after use. Make sure that your friends do not double-dip the wand. Use it once and then throw it away. If you need another layer, use a fresh wand.

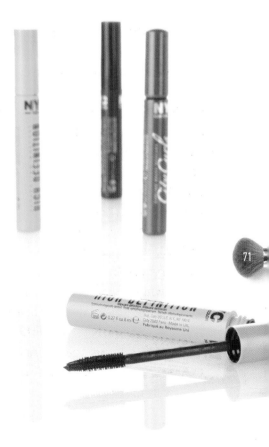

71

There are lots of different types and colours of mascara available:

Black: Gives a defined, dramatic look.

Brown: Creates a softer, more natural look.

Clear: For those who want a completely natural look while defining their eyes.

Colour: For fun, party times!

Waterproof: Does not wash off easily and is great for summer and monsoons. It is the best choice for athletes and swimmers, as it does not melt away with sweat and water. Most water-resistant formulas are so processed that they do not smudge or flake easily.

Water-soluble (non-waterproof): Can be removed easily without the help of eye make-up remover, which means less tugging around your delicate eye area.

A straight brush is good for coating the hard-to-reach corner lashes, while a curved brush makes it easier to coat more of your lashes at once.

How to apply mascara
If you are applying mascara to your bottom lashes, begin with these to prevent the top lashes smudging on your lids.

Next, coat the top lashes, using a zigzag motion from the root to the tip of the lash, to keep them separated. Don't wait for the first coat to dry before applying the next as this will then be likely to clump; instead keep adding new layers while the one before is still wet.

Mascara is the simplest way to define your eyes. You can apply just a touch for a subtle look, or layer it for a more dramatic effect. If you layer two different types of mascara, this helps to create a dramatic effect without making lashes look clumpy.

Tip: Never pump your mascara wand into the tube; when you take the wand out of the tube, twist and pull, and twist as you replace it. Using a pumping action allows air into the tube, which quickly dries out the mascara.

Curling your lashes

If you feel that your eyes could do with an extra boost, try curling your lashes with a pair of eyelash curlers. Do this before you apply your mascara. If you do it afterwards, your lashes will clump together and you could also damage them.

Press the curlers to the roots of your lashes and pump ten times to give a high-definition curl. Apply mascara immediately from the roots to the tips. If you want to apply a second coat, apply it only to the tips of the lashes. If you coat your roots too much you will actually weigh your lashes down, preventing them from curling. Separate your eyelashes with a dry mascara wand to keep them looking natural and soft.

A cautionary tale: when I was 15, heated eyelash curlers were a massive trend. I didn't own any at the time, I only had the traditional metal ones. So I decided to create my own heated version – big mistake! I applied my mascara, waited for it to dry and then heated my metal curlers with a hot hairdryer!

As I clamped down on my eyelashes, not only did I burn my eyelids, but I also melted the mascara and burned straight through my lashes! Devastated, I screamed as I looked at my eyes in the mirror. I had cut off all the lashes of one eye. I never did this again and I'd really like to advise you all that the straightforward unheated metal lash curlers truly are the best way to go.

False lashes

False eyelashes are an amazing way to make your eyes look bigger. The trick is to add a little more of a dramatic effect to your eyes while still looking natural and pretty.

When you are choosing lashes keep in mind their weight. In my experience as a make-up artist, heavy lashes are not only harder to work with but also often

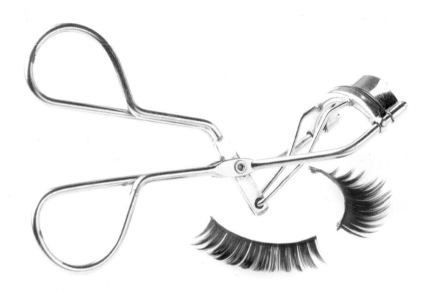

uncomfortable. Look for lightweight lashes which are nice and soft. These can be moulded around your eye, giving perfect definition. They also look like your own lashes and are light as a feather to wear.

Applying the lashes

First curl your natural lashes with eyelash curlers.

Hold the false lashes up to your natural lashes to measure them. If they are too long they will make your eyes look droopy so, if necessary, trim the tips with a small pair of scissors.

Apply false lash glue to the back of your hand and run the edge of your false lashes through it – this avoids any big blobs!

Wait until the lashes feel tacky, or the glue starts turning slightly translucent, and then pop them along the root of your natural lashes (not onto your eyelid!).

Once they are completely dry, wiggle a small amount of mascara through the roots of your own lashes to lift them up and merge them with the false ones. This not only looks more natural but also feels much more comfortable! When it comes to removing the false lashes, you can use eye make-up remover. I would always advise soaking them with a cotton pad first. If you try to pull them off without using anything you could risk pulling out some of your natural lashes! The skin on your eyelids is also very delicate, so treat it kindly.

Extra natural lashes

Opt for individual lashes to give your eyes a fresh, open-eyed, soft look. You can use them all the way along your natural lash line, or just in the outer or inner corners. Use tweezers to apply the lashes as they can be very fiddly! Alternatively, cut your strip lashes in half and use the two outer parts in the outer corners of your eyes.

Individual lashes

Using individual lashes gives you the option of creating the exact volume you desire. I often use individual lashes on brides who would like their eyes to look slightly larger and more emphasised but ultra natural and soft. Some brides just want slightly seductive eyes, in which case I might simply apply a few individual lashes to the outer corners of the natural lashes. Whether you want a full set, or just a few, you apply them in the same way.

The trick to applying them perfectly is to use a pair of tweezers to hold the lash. Hold the centre of the lash to give you more control. Pop a small amount of individual eyelash glue onto the back of your hand and dip the root of the lash into it. Allow a couple of seconds for the glue to become tacky and then place the lash into the root of your own lashes. Continue to add the lashes in this way until you have the effect that you want.

75

Beautiful brows

Our eyebrows frame our faces, and can completely change the way we look. It's very important therefore to get them right. One of the most common mistakes is overplucking of the brows, which take ages to grow back, if ever. If you overpluck you can often end up with patchy brows and a surprised expression! Thin eyebrows are never in fashion for long and are not as flattering as full, feminine, arched brows.

It's well worth having your brows shaped professionally the first time. Beauty therapists have lots of experience and are guaranteed to find your perfect shape. After that if you want to take over and pluck them yourself, you should be able to follow the shape the therapist has given you, plucking away the strays as they grow through. If you pluck them as they grow you won't lose the shape. Leaving them too long may mean you have to start again. Everyone's hair growth rate is different, so you'll need to check regularly in the mirror to judge yours.

The inner edge of each brow should line up with the inner corner of the eye, the arch should be in line with your pupil and the outer edge in line with the outer corner of your eye.

When you are satisfied with the shape, add definition by filling in your brows with a brow powder the same colour as your natural brows. Soft, strong brows are beautiful. Using pencil often creates too much of a hard line, which looks unnatural and harsh. If you like to use pencil because you find it longer lasting, run your eyebrow brush over the tip of the eyebrow pencil to coat the bristles and stroke the brush through your eyebrows gently. Using a brush in this way rather than the tip of the pencil itself creates a much softer, natural fullness and appearance to your brows.

Finish your brows with a brow setting mascara. Run the product up and across through your brows, setting in place any stray hairs. This also helps to keep the definition long lasting.

How to create smoky eyes

With this look you should keep the rest of your make-up as natural as possible, as the focus should be on your eyes.

☐ Prime your eyelids all over, up to your brow bone.

☐ Sweep a light base shadow over your entire lids.

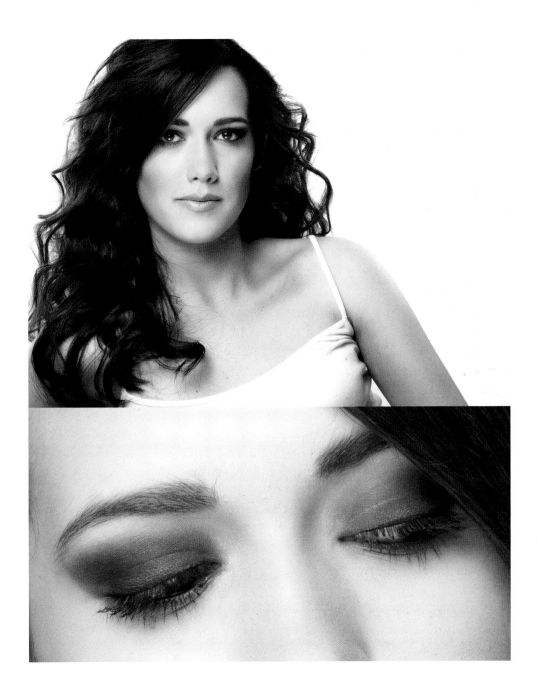

- Smudge a black kohl liner along your top lash line and blend it out over your eyelid.

- Pat a dark shade of shadow on your lower lid, over the eyeliner, from the lash line up to the crease of your eyes, and blend.

- Use a deeper shade layered on top of the first one to give it more intensity.

- Line your top lashes with pencil, gel or liquid liner.

- Smudge a dark kohl pencil along your bottom lash line followed by a dark shadow to make your whole eye look smoky, and finish with three coats of mascara Apply each layer while the previous coat is still wet, to prevent your lashes going clumpy.

> Tip: Layering two different formulas of mascara creates a more dramatic effect.

Fill in your eyebrows with a powder shadow. Powder is fluffy and looks most like natural hair. Pencil can look too hard and harsh. If you have dark eye make-up on, you must make sure your eyebrows don't look too light, otherwise you will lose the dramatic effect. Use an ultra fine, flat eyeliner brush to fill them in, or a ready-made brow brush that comes in some kits.

How to create evening/special occasion eyes

Lots of girls ask me how they can create an evening or special occasion make-up which looks classy, elegant and effortlessly pretty. It's so easy once you know how to do it. In fact it's so simple that you can turn your daytime look to an evening one at your desk and head out straight from work! All you need to do is emphasise your eyes and add a bit of glitz and glam. Here's how I would do it.

Take any colour eyeshadow you like, sweep it over your eyelid and into the

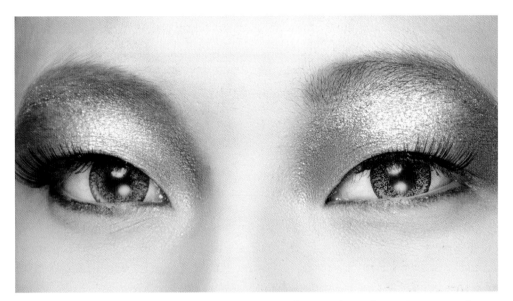

crease of each eye, and blend away the edges. Sweep the colour along your lower lash line. Now blend a darker shade into the crease of your eyelids to give them a real emphasis, and wing the colour out for a flirty appearance. Pat some glitzy shadow over your eyelids to make them sparkle.

Line your upper lashes with a black gel liner and extend it slightly into a small, flirty flick at the outer corners of your eyes. Smudge some black kohl liner along your lower lashes for a mysterious feel. Sweep your mascara from root to tip, up and outwards, to elongate your eyes. Pop on a gloss or lipstick of your choice and you're ready to go!

If you are starting from scratch, the same techniques apply, but make sure you prime your eyelids first to ensure your chosen colour lasts all night.

Tip: If you want dramatic eyes, and would also like dramatic lips, keep your cheeks neutral.

If you're using shimmer, apply it only to one or two features; for example, eyes and lips. Any more than this and you'll glow in the dark! So, if you are using shimmer on cheeks and lips, keep your eyes matt; if you are using shimmer on your eyes and cheeks, keep your lips matt.

How to correct eye shapes

My personal belief is that no matter what their shape, all eyes are beautiful and do not necessarily need correcting. However, make-up helps you to make the best of all your features and below are some tips on how to achieve the most flattering look for your eyes, whatever shape they happen to be.

Close-set eyes (less than one eye's width space between them)

If you have a slender nose, your eyes can often appear close together. You can use eyeshadow to make them look further apart. Use a light base all over your eyelids, up to the brow bone and round to the inner corner of each eye, to make eyes look bright and awake. Use a darker colour in your crease, in a backwards V shape (as shown on page 67), and blend up and out towards the outer corner of each eye. Don't blend the colour towards the inner corners of your eyes as this will close them in again. Keep the colour wide. Apply a little highlighter either side of your nose next to your eyes. Extend the outer corners of your brows with a brow shadow or pencil. If you are wearing eyeliner, start it away from the inner corners of your eyes.

Deep-set eyes

Deep-set eyes recede back into their sockets, so you need to make them more prominent.

Sweep light shadow over the lid, up to the brow bone and into the inner corner of each eye, to brighten them. Use a medium shadow at the outer corners, blend it up and inwards. Keep the lower lid light. If you use eyeliner keep it very thin.

Wide-set eyes (more than one eye's width space between them)

To make eyes appear closer together, apply a medium shadow to the inner half of your eyelid, a lighter shadow on the outer half, and blend. Blend a dark shadow into the crease of each eye towards your nose.

Prominent eyes

These can look as if they are bulging or popping out. To make the eye look less prominent, use a dark shade of eyeshadow near your lash line and over your lower lid, a medium shade for your crease – but don't wing it out, stop at the edge of your eyelid – and a light shadow from the crease to your brow bone. Don't use a dark shadow in the crease as it will make your eyes appear even more prominent. Also, avoid shimmery shadows as these attract the light, again making your eyes appear to pop out more. What you are trying to do is make your eye recede back into its socket.

Hooded eyes

These are sometimes referred to as 'puppy dog eyes'. Use a light shadow all over your eyelid; sweep it up to your brow bone and into the inner corner of each eye. Use a dark shadow over your lower lid and on the outer corner of your eye and sweep up towards your brow bone. Define your eyes with eyeliner top and bottom.

Oval eyes

To make oval eyes appear rounder, apply eyeliner to your top lash line. Beginning at the inner corner of your eye, start with a thin line, thicken it towards the middle, and then make the line thin again at the outer corner.

Round eyes

Extend your eyeliner slightly beyond the outer corner of your eyelid. Sweep a medium colour over your eyelid, into the crease and along your lower lash line. Blend out towards the brow bone to lengthen your eyes.

Almond eyes

Eyes slant slightly upwards at the outer corners. Sweep bold colour or a dark shade over your eyelid, and smudge a medium colour along your lower lash line. Use eyeliner on the outer corner of your eyelid. Apply a lighter or darker shade of eyeshadow and smudge onto the very outer corner of your eye.

Drooping eyes

Eyes slant downwards. Don't use eyeliner beneath your eyes; sweep a light shadow over your eyelids and up to your brow bone. Use a dark or medium shadow in the outer corner of each eyelid and sweep upwards and inwards. If you line your top lid, stop just before the outer corner so that the line doesn't appear to drag your eyes down again.

Play with colour

Fair skin looks gorgeous in cool colours, while the darkest skin tones can look amazing in bright, vibrant shades!

You can apply colour in exactly the same way as I have taught you with first the basic and then the smoky eye; just play and experiment with different shades and colours. You can use lots of different colours together, or stick to one colour in a light, medium and dark shade, or use a light colour with a dark one in your sockets. There are no set rules for applying colour – that's what makes it so much fun to use!

> Tip: Red and pink shades can make your eyes look sore. Blue undertones are the most flattering unless you have a very dark skin tone.

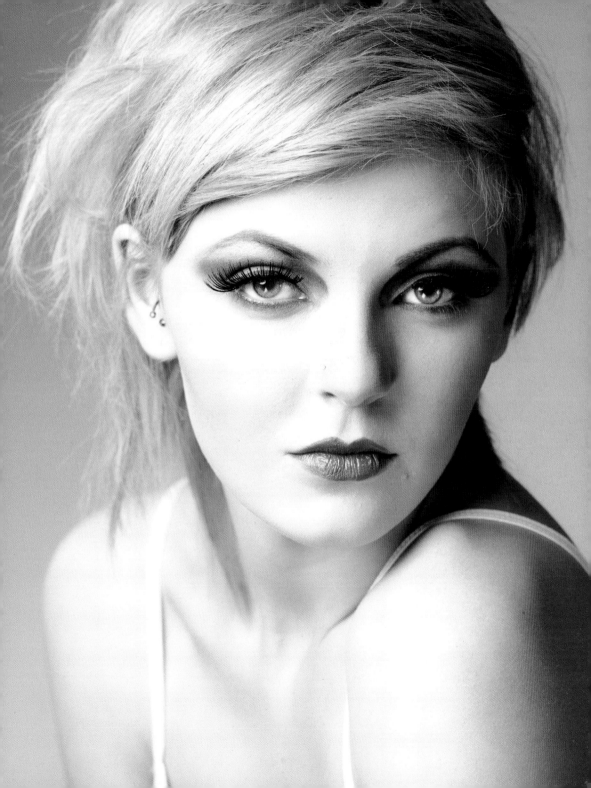

Block colour can look beautiful

Like some of the other looks I've shown you, this is simple but dramatic – really great for a night out.

To achieve this look, prime your eyes with eye primer and then sweep a light base all over your eyelids, up to your brow bone. Pat a purple shadow all over your eyelids and blend it into the crease of each eye, taking care to blend away any hard edges. This look is quite nice if you wing the colour out a little, aiming with your brush towards your temples.

Use your finger to pat a champagne-coloured shimmer onto the centre of your eyelids to give a three-dimensional appearance and to illuminate them. This makes your eyes really dazzling for other people to look at, especially when you're under bright lights or in sunshine.

Keep your skin natural and flawless, with just a hint of warmth, and complete your look with a pretty pink lipstick and a subtle coat of frosted gloss.

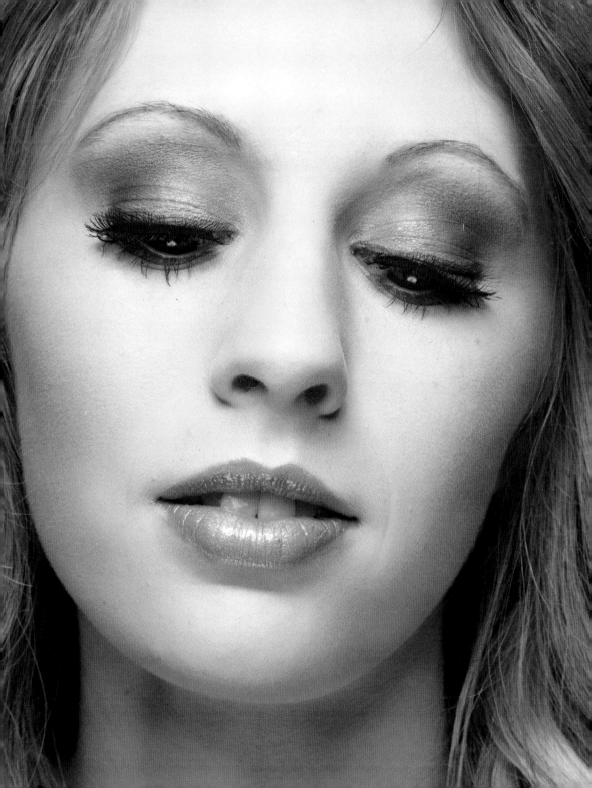

Light can have a transforming effect

As I mentioned earlier in the book, when I was training as a make-up artist I had a fear of colour and of going too bold. Every look I created appeared natural, even if it wasn't meant to. So my tutor set me the task of achieving dramatic, bright make-up, with the aim of moving me out of my comfort zone. It worked. I realised just how amazing and how much fun colour can be!

The trick to judging how dramatic you can go with your make-up is to understand the light around you. Lighting makes a huge impact on the way your make-up looks. Have you ever found that it appears different in every mirror that you peer into? The reason that we go lighter with our make-up during the day, and bolder at night, is because sunlight is one of the strongest light forms there is. While studio lights drown out colour, sunlight emphasises everything and is much less forgiving. Evening sunlight is softer, with a golden glow. It is said that the light is most beautiful at this time. At night and in the winter we rely on man-made lighting, which enables us to go much wilder with colour.

However, to this day I still believe that learning to perfect natural-looking make-up before moving on to high-fashion drama helped me to become a successful make-up artist. This is because I am able to apply make-up in such a way that my model's skin looks flawless and natural, even when the result is a super high-fashion look.

Again, I want to stress that going bold with your make-up isn't about plastering it on; it is about emphasising your features to a greater extent than you normally would. I am of the opinion that make-up should always look like real skin, whatever style you are aiming for. If you can keep this in mind, no matter how bold a statement you make with your eyes and lips, it will never look over the top, as long as it is applied correctly.

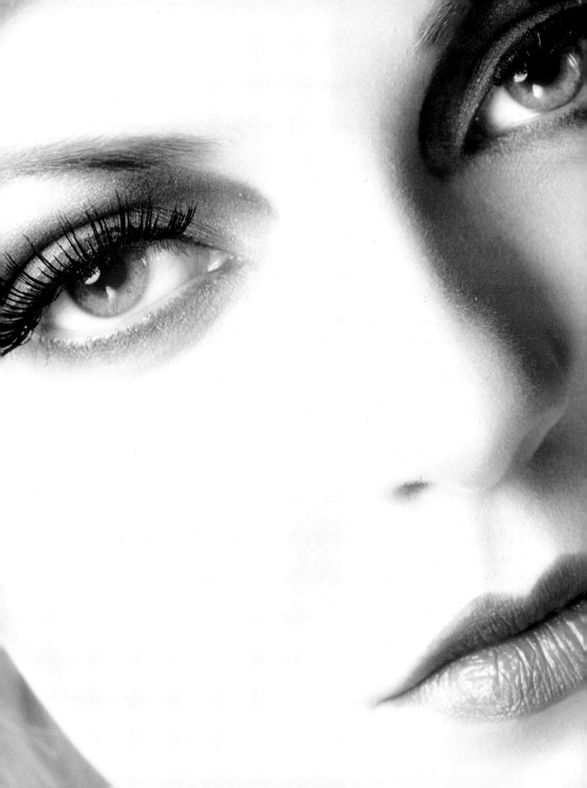

Metallic colours can look stunning

If you want a really dramatic, bold eye colour, wet your brush, dip it into your eyeshadow and sweep it all over your lower eyelids. If you use this technique with metallic colours, you can achieve a tinfoil effect! Try it with metallic gold and silver – the results are amazing.

If you don't feel too confident about experimenting with this look, try it out on the back of your hand first to see what you think.

Try playing with the tinfoil effect. I chose silver for the look shown here because it is stunning against Hayley's fair skin and honey-coloured hair, but you can use any colour you like.

Apply an eye primer all over your eyelids and up to your brow bone. Next pat a silver cream shadow over your eyelids and use a fluffy brush to blend the colour into the crease of each eye. If you take the silver slightly above the crease of your eyes it will give the look more drama. Keep your lower lash line free of eyeshadow to maintain the emphasis on your eyelids, but apply mascara to your top and bottom lashes to prevent the make-up from looking top heavy.

Buff a peach blusher over the apples of your cheeks to warm your complexion against the colder silver. Team the look with apricot lipstick finished with an apricot gloss.

Use colour as eyeliner

I love simple make-up that makes a statement. I often find it looks the most beautiful, because it isn't confusing; it says effortlessly pretty and right on trend. If we use colour everywhere sometimes we don't know where to look first.

When you look at the photo of model Hayley, you are instantly drawn to her eyes. The turquoise liner is bright and captivating, but at the same time, simple, fun and pretty. You could use this technique with any colour.

To create Hayley's look, first prime your eyes with eye primer and then sweep a natural, matt shadow over your eyelids up to your brow bone. Dip a fine eyeliner brush into a little eyeliner sealer, cover it in a turquoise eyeshadow and then draw a line along your top lash line. Alternatively, you can buy aqua colour eyeshadows;

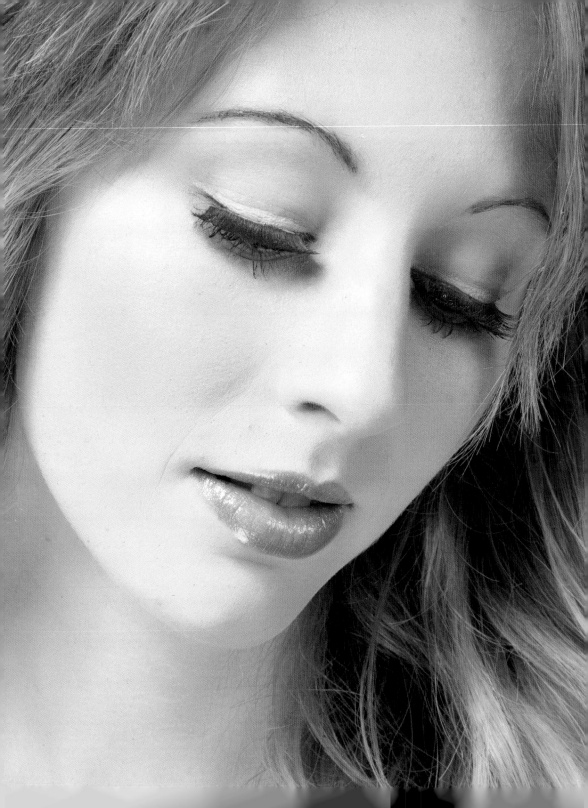

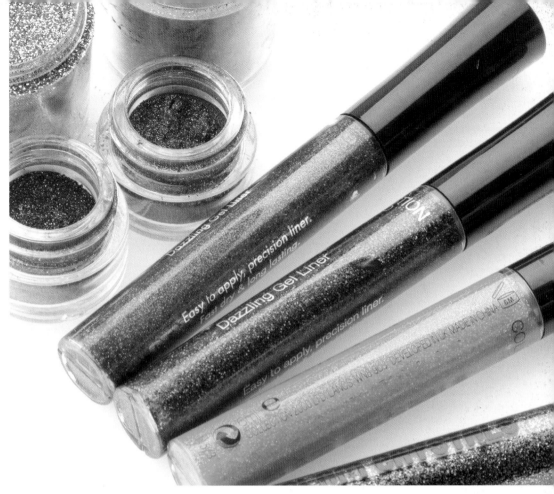

you dip your brush in water and use the same technique. Keep your lower lash line clear and fresh, so that the emphasis is on the bright colour.

The rest of your make-up should look very natural; just pop a little peachy blusher over the apples of your cheeks and apply lip colour similar to your own natural colour, topped with a coat of gloss for a healthy shine.

You can also buy ready-made colour and glitter eyeliners. These can be applied as eyeliner, or you can pat them all over your eyelid for a glittery sparkle that will stay put all day. Line your eyes with glitter gel liner and then pat it over your eyelids while it is still wet.

Glitter looks beautiful on anyone. Try sweeping it over eyes and cheeks for a fabulous party look!

CHAPTER 5

Pretty Lips

My top secret tip for soft, pretty lips

Keep them moisturised all the time. During the day wear a lip balm with SPF underneath your lip gloss or lipstick. At night, dot a small amount of extra virgin olive oil onto your lips and massage it in. It acts as a completely natural lip balm and is one of the most nourishing products that I have found! Once a week, using circular motions, rub a sugar scrub into your lips to remove any dead skin cells and stop lips looking dry or flaky. (This tastes really yummy, too; I recommend strawberry.) You can also gently rub your toothbrush over your lips to get the same result.

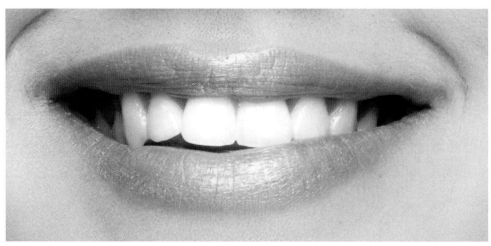

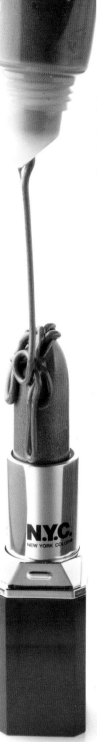

Lipstick formulas

There are lots of different lipstick products to choose from. My favourites are glossy lipsticks that give you a really healthy shine. When I'm applying lipstick I always add a sweep of gloss on top to keep my lips feeling moist. I guess it all comes down to your own personal preference.

There are plenty of long-lasting products on the market, but I find they really dry out your lips; later in this chapter you'll find my tips and tricks to help you get the same result.

Below are some of the most popular lipstick products

☐ **Matt lipstick**

☐ **Glossy lipstick**

☐ **Lip stain**

☐ **Lip pencils**

☐ **Lip liner**

☐ **Lip balm**

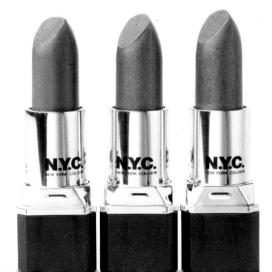

93

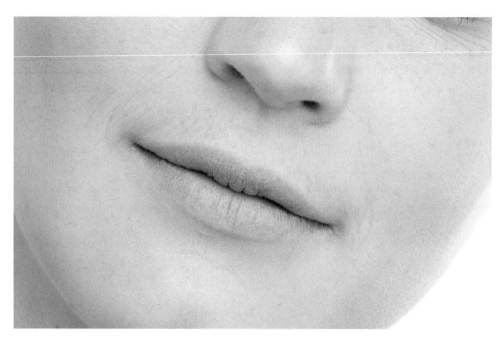

Choosing your lip colour

Do you ever wonder which colour lipstick suits you best?

When you are testing out lip colours at the make-up counters, test them on the tips of your fingers; the skin colour here is nearer to the natural colour of your lips than is the skin on the back of your hand. Hold your fingers next to your lips and see which colour you feel makes you shine.

- **Pale lips:** These suit pastel shades, such as beige, dusty pink, light coral, pale pink and bright red.

- **Medium lips:** Go for brown, rose, pink, orange and warm red.

- **Dark/very red lips:** Opt for brown, deep red, plum, deep chocolate, deep berry.

Your perfect, natural shade of lipstick will be a close match to the natural tone of your lips. One shade darker or one shade lighter will always look flattering too.

Tips for choosing red lipstick

Did you know that wearing red actually boosts your confidence?

If you have dark skin, choose lipstick with orange or brown undertones.

Light skin tones look better with colder, intense shades of red.

If your teeth look yellow against a red lipstick, you have the wrong colour!

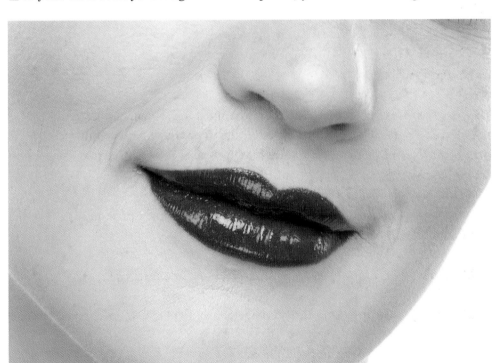

95

How to apply your lipstick

Believe it or not, there is an art to applying lipstick. Your lips, like your eyes, are a very powerful feature, so I'm going to share my tips and tricks for a perfect pout.

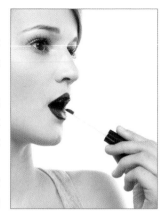

Massage some lip balm into your lips before you apply anything else, to keep them soft and plump. Blot your lips with a tissue to remove the excess so that your lipstick stays put and doesn't rub straight off.

Begin with a lip liner, even if you are going to wear lip gloss. Choose a shade that matches either your natural lip colour or the colour of the lipstick or gloss that you are going to wear.

Draw around your lips perfectly, exactly on the lip line. You can go slightly outside or inside your lip line to make lips look fuller or thinner, but not too much or you will look like a drag queen! If you don't fancy using a coloured lip liner, try a skin-toned highlighting one. This will emphasise your lips as the light catches it and you won't see any hard lines.

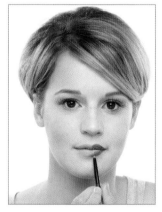

Lightly fill in the rest of your lips with the liner and blend it in, as this helps to make your lipstick or gloss last longer and blends away any hard lines. If you find that your lipstick often wears off quickly, try using a lip stain underneath it.

If you are going to wear lipstick, apply it over the top of your lip liner, right into the corners of your mouth, and then blot your lips with a tissue. Finish with a small sweep of lip gloss to stop your lips feeling dry. Or, if you want matt lips, dust some powder over your lipstick to create a velvety pout.

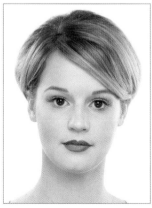

Have fun with your lip colour; vivid lips say

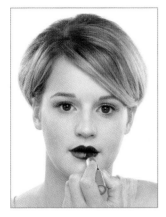

personality and confidence! If there is a bright shade that you love, but you don't want it to look too over the top, you can tone it down a bit. First, apply lip balm or Vaseline to your lips and then – using a lip brush – add a small amount of colour and blend it in.

If you don't like wearing lipstick or gloss, try a lip stain. This gives colour to your lips but dries instantly so that you don't feel as if you are wearing anything. It also looks great with a slick of clear lip gloss over the top if you want a dewy effect.

Lip tips
Create full lips

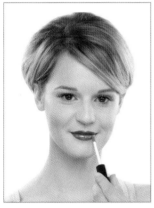

Use a lip liner to widen the middle of your top and bottom lips. Use light or medium shades of lipstick and dot some gloss or a highlighter on the middle of your bottom lip to make it look fuller. Take your lip gloss right out to the edges of your lips to highlight them and make them look fuller. Pop some highlighter along your cupid's bow, to emphasise the curvy area. You can also experiment with lip plumping products. Make sure your lips are completely moisture free before you put it on, so that you get the best results.

Make your lips thinner

Personally, I love full lips but if you do want to make yours appear thinner, use darker shades of lipstick and make sure you don't line over the edges of your lips. This will give an illusion of smaller lips.

Natural, unmade-up lips

This is my favourite look for lips because it makes you look really healthy and radiant. There are different ways of achieving natural, unmade-up lips. I tend to skip lip liner and use lipstick as a stain. I apply the lipstick to my finger and then pat it onto my lips, taking it right up to the edge of my lip line, especially around the cupid's bow. This makes my lips look fuller. Choose a shade close to your natural lip tone.

You can also buy commercial lip stains, which are specifically designed not to budge. The nice thing about lip stains is that even as they do start to wear off they still look lush!

Another trick is to apply a natural liner to the edges of your lips and smudge it with your finger or a brush to fill in the rest of your lips. Finally, pop some gloss or lip balm over the top.

Long-lasting lip colour

The staying power of lip colours tends to vary depending on the person. My lipstick might last all day, while other people have to reapply theirs every 20 minutes! It all depends on how moist your lips are, how often you lick or chew them, how often you eat and drink.

Here are a few tricks to make it last longer.

☐ Use your lip liner all over your lips underneath your lipstick or gloss.

☐ Choose a matt lipstick as it may last longer than a glossy one.

☐ Use a lip stain.

☐ Apply powder between coats of lipstick.

CHAPTER 6

Play with your Looks

I meet so many girls who say to me, 'I'm stuck in a make-up rut; I've worn my make-up the same way every day since I began wearing it. How can I change it?'

My answer is always, 'Experiment; keep an eye on how fashion trends change. Grab all your magazines and practise recreating some of the looks in there.'

If you follow this advice you'll have loads of fun and you'll soon be confident about changing your make-up whenever you feel like it, and daring to go from simple to bold, bright and colourful. Invite a group of friends over, get your make-up out and have fun trying out different looks on each other.

To get you started, I have created some looks for you to practise with. Once you have mastered them, be daring, swap colours around, mix looks together, be *you*!

Bare eyes & bright lips

This is by far one of my favourite looks – elegant yet striking. It enhances your natural beauty but adds a twist of fun too. The fashion catwalks and retail clothes shops alike are inspired by past fashions that are given a modern edge in contemporary surroundings. Make-up is inspired in much the same way. Bare eyes and bright lips hold a hint of the 1950s, when the gorgeous Marilyn Monroe sported natural eyes, dramatic eyeliner and bright red lips.

I've modernised the look on Bethany Rose, with shimmery shadows, rosy pink cheeks and bright pink lip colour. I have also applied false lashes for extra effect.

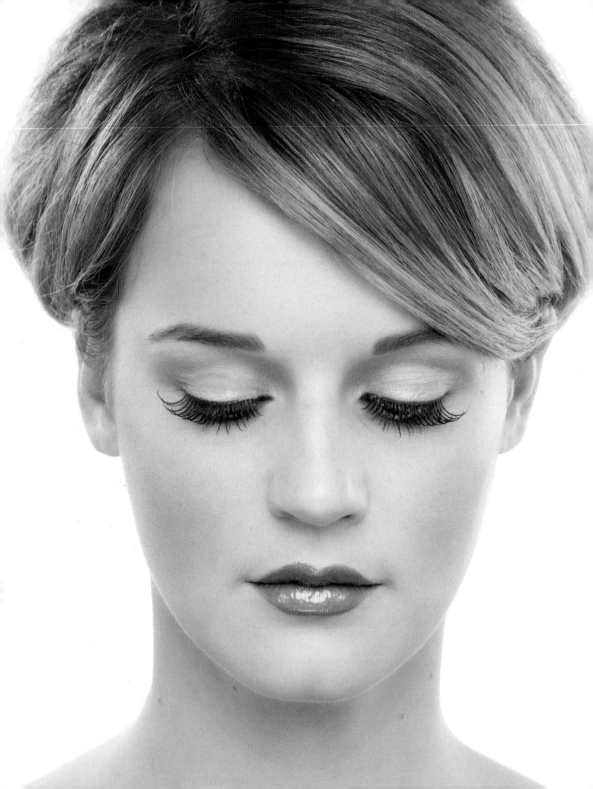

If you want to recreate this fabulous look, first apply an eye primer and then sweep a light shimmery eyeshadow base all over your eyelids and up to your brow bone. Give your skin warmth with a dusting of bronzer over the apples of your cheeks, forehead, nose, neck and chin. Smile and sweep a baby pink blusher over the apples of your cheeks and blend it up towards your temples.

For this look I applied some light, natural false lashes to the roots of Bethany's own lashes and then followed with lashings of mascara to her top and bottom lashes. You can do the same if you would like a little extra emphasis on your eyes.

Run a very fine line of dark brown eyeliner along the roots of your lashes to give extra depth, but keep your bottom lash line clear. Finally, line your lips with a natural lip liner and then apply a spot of bright pink lipstick and a dash of gloss to your lips. Remember, you can use any brightly coloured lipstick for this elegant look.

1950s modern beauty

As a make-up artist, one of the looks I am most often asked to recreate is that of the 1950s, inspired by glamorous screen goddesses like Marilyn Monroe and Sophia Loren – both exquisitely beautiful women. What I like about these women though is that, despite their uncommon beauty, they still looked like real women – pretty, curvy and natural.

In the 1950s make-up made a statement; it was simple, but bold and beautiful. I'm going to show you how you can recreate this glamorous look for yourself.

Prime your skin and apply your foundation in the areas where you need it. Dust a translucent powder lightly over your skin. The 1950s complexion was fairly matt; however, the trend in modern make-up is for a dewy, healthy look, so don't go too crazy with your powder, your aim is radiant skin.

Skip the bronzer and reach for a peachy pink blusher. Buff this over the apples of your cheeks and sweep it up towards your temples for a soft, subtle glow.

With this look, eyes and lips are your statement features, and eyeliner was a big part of the 1950s style.

Prime your eyelids and sweep a light, matt shadow over the top of your primer. If you want an extra modern look you could swap the matt eyeshadow for

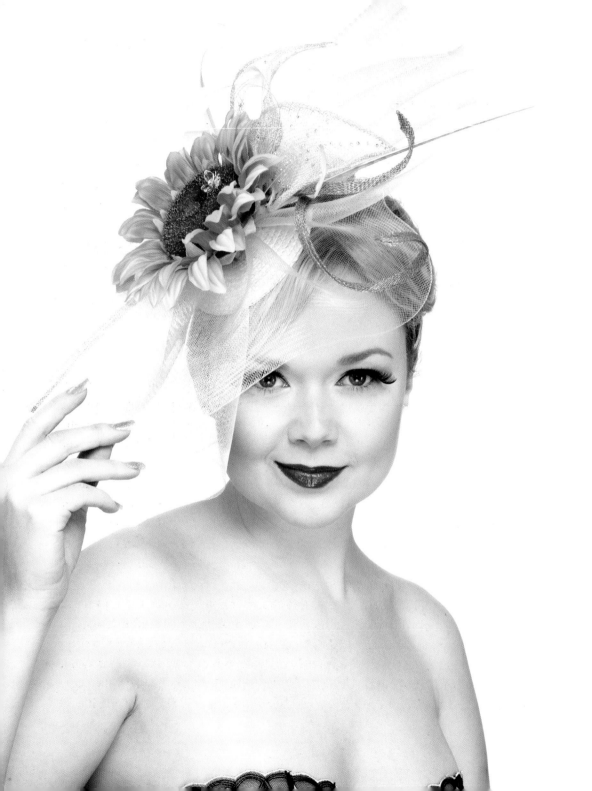

a shimmery or frosted one.

Shade your creases ever so lightly with a medium shade of shadow in beige-brown or bronze.

Line your top lashes with black gel liner as this gives a very defined, smooth result. Begin at the inner corner of each eye with a very fine line, make it thicker towards the middle, and taper off again towards the outer corners. Flick it out slightly at the outer corners.

Apply false lashes for more drama and keep your lower lash line completely clear; perhaps add some mascara to maintain balance. Define your eyebrows. In the 1950s eyebrows were thick, dark and feminine.

Line your lips with red lip liner and fill them in. Apply red lipstick: matt for a more vintage look, or glossy for a modern twist.

A hint of vamp

The vampy, effortlessly pretty look is one that has been on trend for some time now. Gone are the days of the set hairdo and precise, heavy make-up. Today it's more about boho chic like Sienna Miller's loose waves and natural, unmade-up face, and Kate Moss's rock chick style. The aim is to look as though you can achieve this yourself with the minimum of fuss.

I chose to recreate this feel with model Emily. Her hairstyle is very modern, chic and elegant, falling softly around her face. Her features are soft but played up, really showing them at their best. Here's how you can achieve Emily's look.

Prime your skin and buff your foundation into the areas where it is needed. Remember, your skin doesn't need to look completely masked; the point of this look is to let your natural beauty glow through.

Prime your eyelids and apply a light shimmer shadow over the top of the primer, up to your brow bone. Apply a slate cream shadow over your lower lids and stop at the crease; you don't want the colour to go above it. Pat a frosted silver shadow over the top of the cream shadow and sweep it over your lower lash line.

Apply a black gel liner along your top lash line from the inner to the outer corners of your eyes. Smudge the liner gently while it is still wet, to soften it, and

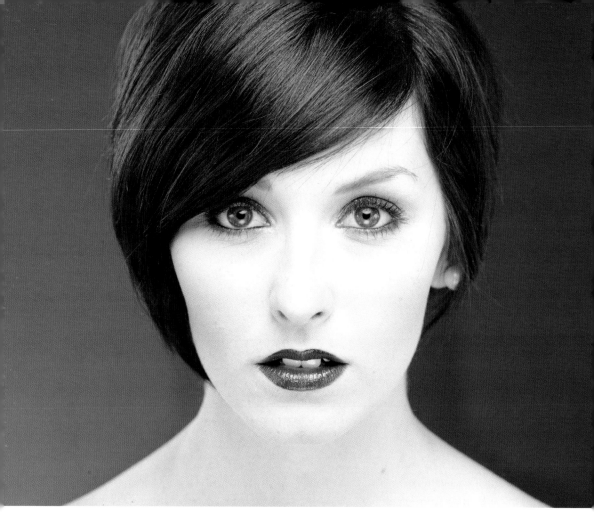

then smudge kohl liner along your lower lashes from outer to inner corners. Run some black kohl liner along your water line (the inside rim of your eyes). Zigzag your mascara wand from the roots of your lashes to the tips, focusing more heavily on the roots to give your lashes more definition, and keeping the tips softer.

You want a fresh and pretty feel with this make-up: vamp chic, not vampire. Cheeks should be soft; contour your cheekbones lightly with bronzer and then dust a light coat of pinky blusher over them.

Use a plum red on your lips. Use your finger or a lip brush to smudge it into your lips, and tidy the edges with a lip liner. Don't try to make it too perfect; this look always looks nice if it's a little edgy.

Colourful & smoky eyes

Smoky eyes are a much-loved trend that reaches right back through the decades, changing slightly from one era to the next, but never seeming to go out of fashion. It's a look that's so much fun to create – you can use all sorts of colours and blend them together for some really pretty alternatives to the traditional dark, smoky eye.

Simply by playing with colours you can completely change the feel of the smoky eye look. Dark, smoky eyes are powerful, strong and confident; pretty pastels are soft and alluring.

Apply coloured smoky eyeshadow in the same way as a neutral or dark smoky eye make-up. To create Natalie's gorgeous pastel eyes, shown here, first prime your eyelids with eye primer all the way up to your brow bone.

Next, sweep a light, shimmery eyeshadow base all over your eyelids and, again, right up to your brow bone.

Pat a light shade of purple (lilac) over your eyelids, finishing at the crease of each eye. Using a medium shade of purple, draw a backwards V onto the outer edges of your lower lids. Next use your fluffy eyeshadow brush to blend the colour into the crease of each eye, making them smoulder, blending the colour towards the inner corners of your eyes and leaving a highlighted space in the centre of your lower eyelid.

Using the same shade of medium purple, smudge it along your lower lashes. Use your fluffy eyeshadow brush to blend a lighter shade of purple into the crease of each eye, and blend until all the lines are invisible and the colour looks as if it is fading out.

Apply black kohl liner to the roots of your lashes top and bottom and smudge it, using an eyeshadow brush, to make it look smoky. Sweep an intense-volume black mascara into your lashes top and bottom.

Finish the look with a peach gloss lipstick and a sweep of peach blusher over the apples of your cheeks and up towards your temples.

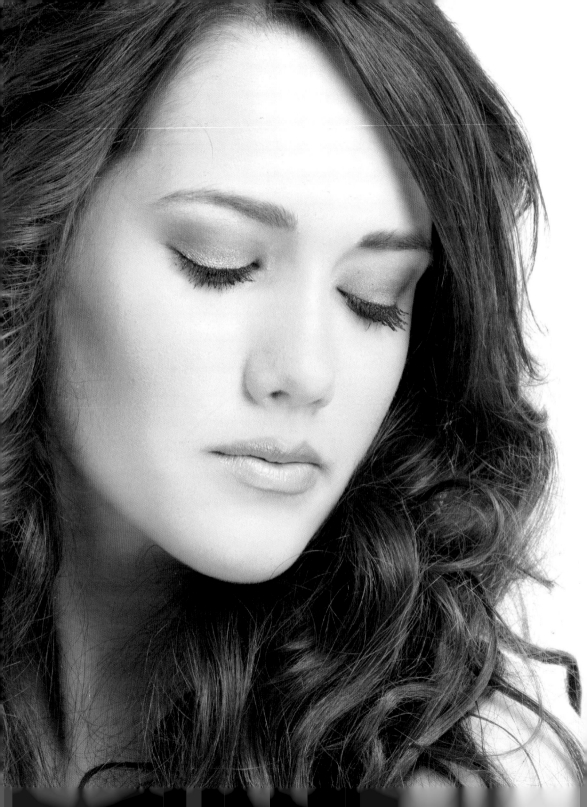

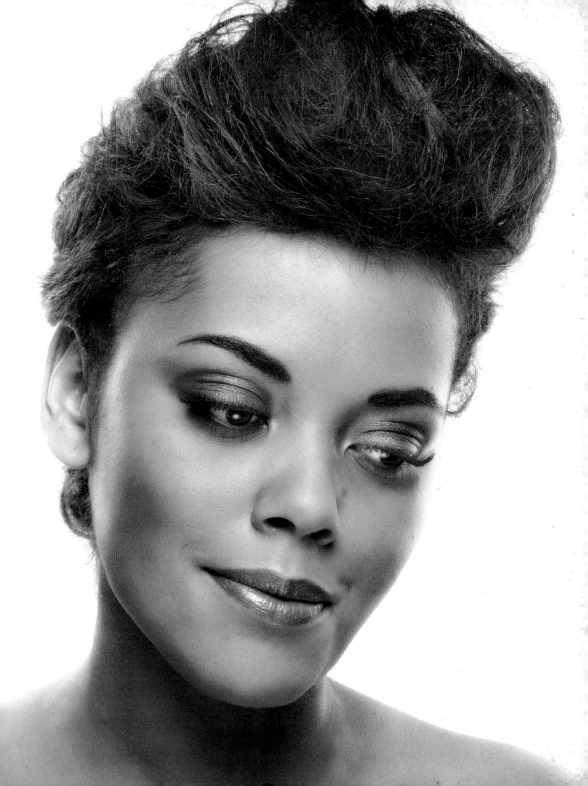

Bold & colourful eyes

It's easy to get stuck in a rut with our make-up, so keep your creative spark flying and experiment with different colours and techniques in applying your eyeshadow.

Florence has beautiful, golden skin, so I wanted to use some gorgeous vibrant colours to complement it. Not many skin tones can get away with hot pink eyeshadow, but because golden skins have yellow undertones (rather than pink), the colour can actually be flattering.

The smoky eye is seen everywhere, so I want to show you a unique look that you can play around with in your own way. This is an example of how you can really have fun with your eye make-up.

Prime your eyes with an eye primer and then sweep a light golden, shimmery shadow all over your eyelids and up to your brow bone. Apply a cream shadow to your eyelids and then, using an eyeshadow brush, gently pat a hot pink shadow over the top of it, following the shape of your socket line. Keep the lines fairly sharp and bold.

Apply an electric blue shadow to the outer corners of your eyes and then use your fluffy eyeshadow brush to blend the two colours together slightly, where they meet. Apply the same electric blue shadow along your lower lash line.

Finally, using your fluffy eyeshadow brush, blend the edges ever so slightly to soften any harsh-looking areas.

I used natural false lashes on Florence to give her look more drama, followed by a light coat of mascara on both her top and bottom lashes. Again, false lashes are optional; it depends on whether or not you like wearing them.

Natural & pretty day look

Sometimes we just want to look effortlessly natural and pretty. This can seem to be the most challenging look to accomplish because we want to look flawless while appearing to be wearing no make-up. (It's easy once you know how.)

Here I have created for Chloe a naturally pretty, girl-next-door look and I am going to show you how you can create this look yourself.

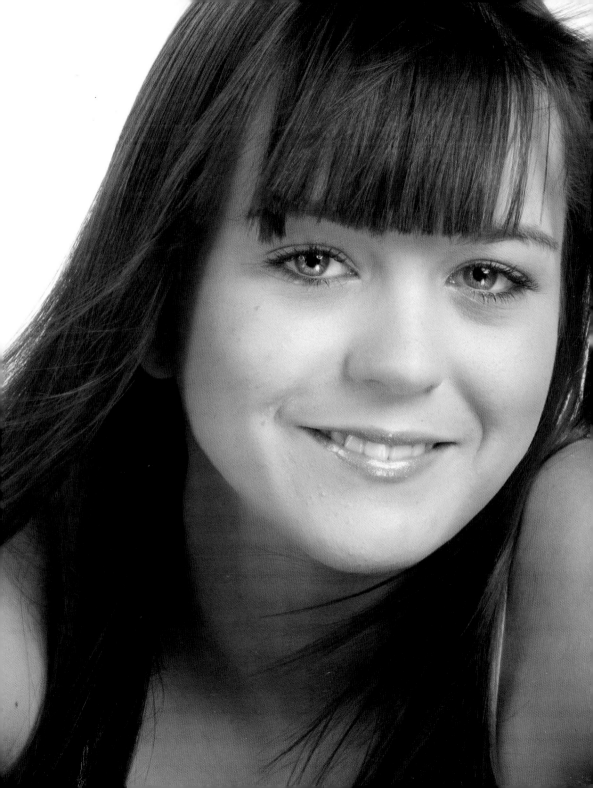

Stick to flesh-tone colours on your eyes, lips and cheeks. Apply a lightweight liquid foundation with a multi-use foundation brush and buff it over your skin gently to give your face a flawless but barely there complexion. Literally all you want to do is even out your skin tone.

Pop some bronzer onto the apples of your cheeks, followed by a sweep of baby pink blusher. Sweep this up towards your temples and blend until there are no lines.

Apply your eye primer and then pat a light eyeshadow base all over your eyelids and up to your brow bone, then apply a light peach, shimmery eyeshadow all over your eyelids and blend it into the crease of each eye. Make sure that all edges of your make-up are perfectly blended. Smudge a darker brown into the outer corner of your lower lash line to define your eyes.

Apply mascara to your top and bottom lashes and finish with pretty pink lips in a baby pink gloss.

Bronzed goddess

The summer sun rolls in and out of season but the bronzed goddess in you doesn't have to follow it. If you love that tanned beach babe look, I can show you exactly how to achieve it all year round!

The key to this look is gorgeous, glowing simplicity. You want healthy, dewy, bronzed skin, teamed with fresh, wide-awake eyes. Summer is all about looking and feeling happy and refreshed, and this is what you are aiming to to reflect with your make-up.

Begin by blending an illuminated tinted moisturiser into your skin to give your face a radiant glow; pay particular attention to the areas of your face that you want to highlight. For Hayley's look, shown here, I used a dewy liquid-to-powder make-up in areas that needed more coverage and an under eye perfecter one shade lighter than her foundation beneath her eyes to make them bright and fresh.

Next I contoured Hayley's cheekbones using a slightly darker shade of foundation in the hollows of her cheeks, blending seamlessly. I then blended a small amount of pinky-peach cream blush over her cheekbones, followed by a

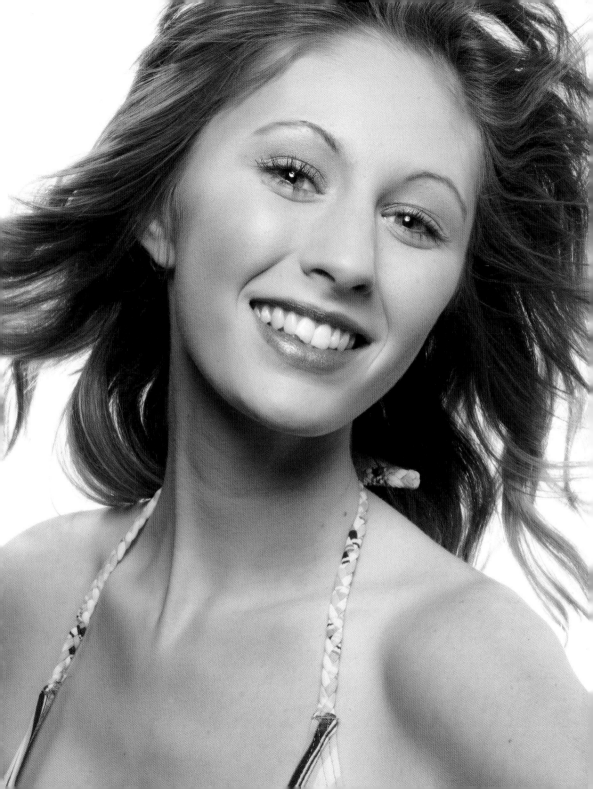

highlighter along the tops of the cheekbones.

I dusted a very fine layer of translucent powder over Hayley's face to set the make-up. And then, using a fluffy bronzer brush, I swept a bronze glow over the apples of her cheeks, forehead, nose, chin, neck and eyelids – everywhere the sun would naturally hit.

I used my fingers to apply a very light gold cream shadow to her eyelids, and then, using a fluffy brush, swept a small amount of bronze pigment over her eyelids, slightly up into the crease of each eye and along the lower lash line. I then applied mascara to her top and bottom lashes.

I completed the look with a bronze lipstick. Using my finger I patted the colour into her lips and then finished with a slick of shimmery gloss.

CHAPTER 7

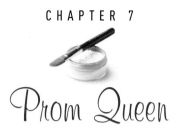

Prom Queen

Sparkling, rosy and radiant

Prom night is a big time for celebration. You've spent years working hard at your education and now it's time to party!

But this isn't just any party; it symbolises the start of your journey towards becoming an adult, so you definitely want to dazzle. Just as a bride waits so long for her big day, so do young girls seem to wait for ever for theirs! I think it's just as important to sparkle on your prom night as it is on your wedding day. So let's direct as much energy into making you look radiant as you have put into all your hard work at school or uni!

Prep at least a week before the prom night.

- [ ] Exfoliate your skin – a gentle face scrub for your complexion and a body scrub for your body.
- [ ] Use a face mask once at the beginning of the week of the prom.
- [ ] Moisturise your body and face every day.
- [ ] Get some great beauty sleep – at least eight hours a night, if you can!
- [ ] Drink lots of water – up to eight glasses a day – to keep you looking hydrated and radiant.
- [ ] If you're going to have a fake tan, exfoliate the night before. Give yourself a trial spray tan a few weeks before your prom; if you don't like it, there's time for it

to fade. If you do like it, have the spray two or three days before your prom. The first day it always looks really bright, but by the second day it will have settled into your skin's natural colour.

- Remove all traces of your make-up every night and let your skin breathe.
- Use plenty of lip balm every day – dry, cracked lips are never a hot look!
- If you get pimples don't squeeze them.
- Tell yourself you have a picture-perfect complexion!

Prom make-up

Here's how to get Hannah's look: prep your skin with a skin primer to give you a silky smooth complexion and to make sure that your make-up will last all through a long night of energetic dancing!

Use a fluffy multi-use foundation brush to apply an illuminated tinted moisturiser to your cheeks, forehead, nose, chin and collarbones. Buff your foundation into areas of your face that need more coverage.

Use your fingers to pat a small amount of under eye corrector beneath your eyes to lighten and brighten them. It's really important for this look to appear radiant and glowing; spring fresh, but with hints of summer too.

Sweep a peachy bronzer over the apples of your cheeks, forehead, nose, chin, neck and eyelids. Do this very softly, to give your complexion warmth with a subtle glow.

Buff apricot blusher over the apples of your cheeks and up over your cheekbones. Apply an eye primer to your eyelids to ensure that the colour stays crease free and in place.

Next use a very light gold, shimmery shadow over your eyelids and sweep it up to your brow bone.

Use an eyeshadow brush to pat a shimmery green shadow over your eyelids and then use an eyeshadow blending brush to blend the colour into the crease of each eyelid. Sweep the green slightly along your lower lash line. Apply a very thin line of eyeliner to the roots of your upper lashes and keep your lower lashes bare.

Finish your eye make-up by softly applying coats of mascara to your top and bottom lashes. Comb through them with a clean, dry mascara wand, to keep them soft and natural.

Tidy your brows with a soft brow shadow and fix them gently by combing through them with a clear eyebrow gel. This will fix any stray hairs and leave you with perfectly shaped brows to frame your face.

Finally, apply an apricot gloss to your lips to give you a pretty pout.

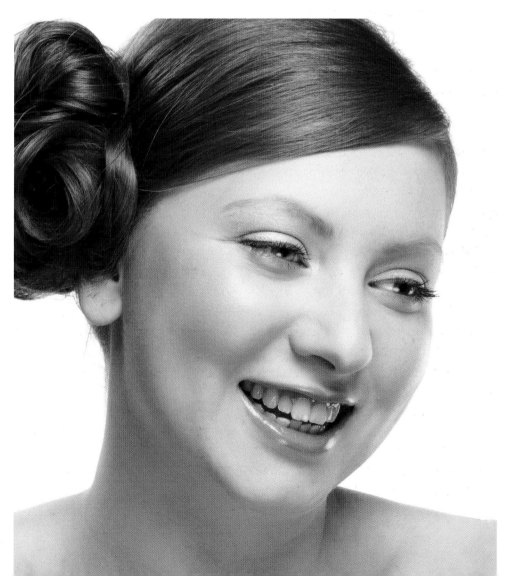

CHAPTER 8

Party Girl

Party make-up

Party time is crazy make-up time! For me, much of the fun of a night out comes from the time beforehand, when I'm getting ready! One of the things I enjoy most is getting the girls round and glamming up together. I find that we all give each other superconfidence in both our clothes and our looks.

There are so many looks you can play with depending on what you choose to wear. Your clothes and make-up express who you really are, in your own time, when you let your hair down. So get creative and have fun!

If I am wearing something bold and bright I often opt for minimal make-up, with nude eyes and bright lips. If I am wearing dark or light colours I like to emphasise my eyes. One of my favourite looks though is glitzy, because it's fun. If you're wearing black it's an awesome way of jazzing it up. This is the look I chose to give model Florence, and here's how you can achieve it.

Sweep an eye primer all over your eyelids and up to your brow bone, and then pat a metallic gold cream eyeshadow all over your eyelids and blend it into the crease of each eye. Before you apply glitter, dust some loose powder beneath your eyes to catch any that might fall onto your skin. Use your eyeshadow brush to pat loose gold eye glitter all over your lower eyelids and into the crease of each eye. Apply mascara to your top and bottom lashes and tidy your eyebrows with a fine brush and brow shadow.

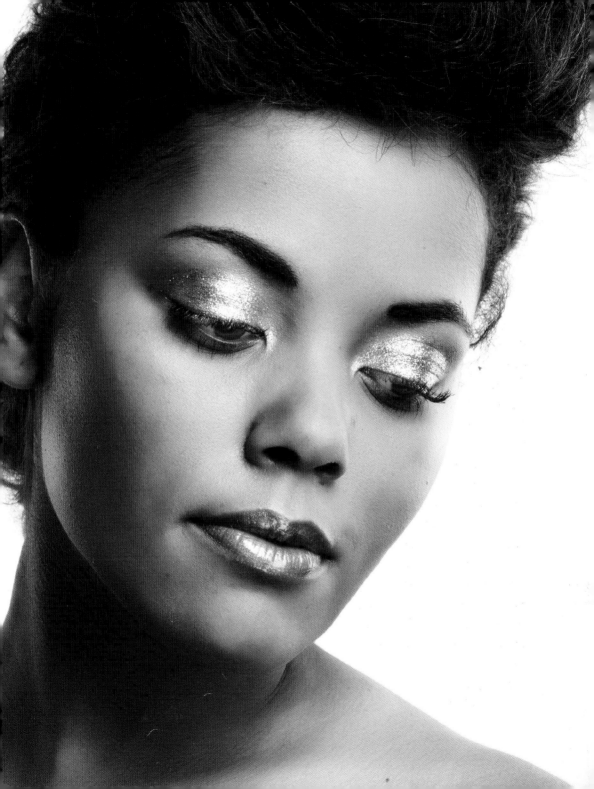

Complete the look by sweeping a peach blusher over the apples of your cheeks, and applying a peachy pink lip gloss generously to your lips.

> **Tip:** eye gloss or eye glitter glue (specifically made for your eyes) is fab for making your glitter stay put.

Match your make-up to your party clothes

The first rule for party make-up is to colour match your complexion, *not* your clothes. For example, you may be wearing an orange top but this doesn't necessarily mean that you can pull off a bright orange lipstick. Instead, think shades: choose the shade of lipstick that best suits you and go from there.

Matching your make-up to your party clothes is seriously great fun. Identical colour matching is totally dated, so if you have a navy blue dress, don't feel that you have to team it with a pair of navy blue peepers!

The awesome thing about today's fashion is that it is completely unique. If you walk into Top Shop you will see an astonishing array of colour: greens with purples, yellows with camel and terracotta, even pink with orange – and at one time that was one of the biggest fashion faux pas of all!

Today pretty much anything goes, as long as you wear your shades right. Your colours need to complement each other. For example, on model Hannah I used green eyeshadow teamed with apricot lips (see page 115). Green and orange are complementary colours on the colour wheel and therefore look great together.

When choosing your colours, hold them up against your skin and the clothes you are going to wear. If the colours look good together and create a glow, you've got it right. If they look muddy or sallow next to each other they are a no-no together. If you can't decide, ask someone else's advice; friends and family are usually happy to help.

CHAPTER 9

Pre-teen Princess

Make-up tips

The pre-teen years are a fantastic time. You may feel like the baby of the family, or wish you could be like your big sister, but, believe me, this is is one of the loveliest times of your life. You can be a princess! This is the age for fun, so invite your friends round and just play with colour and glitter!

Girls under 13 most definitely should not be wearing foundation. If you have any blemishes you want to cover, use a small foundation or concealer stick on the blemish only. If you have very dark under eyes, you can use a small amount of light-reflective corrector.

Other than that, just apply a pop of pinky blusher to your cheeks, and some shimmer or colour eyeshadow to your eyes. Finish with a sweep of colouredl or sparkly lip gloss. You don't need to use lip liner.

Just to remind you how beautiful a make-up-free face can look, model Katherine, pictured here, is wearing absolutely no make-up!

119

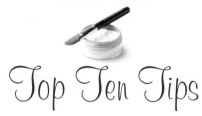

CHAPTER 10

Top Ten Tips

1. **Be Confident, be unique, be real, be you** – don't worry about what other people think; what counts is what you like. Personality is everything, so let it shine through.

2. **Learn to love the way you look** – if you do, so will others, and you'll be surprised how quickly you settle into your own skin and see your confidence grow.

3. **Have fun with your looks, experiment and discover** – you are only young once.

4. **Understand and look after your skin, your health, your body and your mind** – if you look after yourself now you'll be beautiful for ever.

5. **Remember that celebrities are real people too** – just like you or me.

6. **Foundation is designed to match and even out our skin tone, not to tan us** – use bronzer to add colour.

7. **Make-up is designed to make us look pretty, not plastered.**

8. **Our eyelashes are meant to look soft, striking and pretty** – avoid spider leg lashes!

9. **Always, always take off your make-up at bedtime!**

10. **Remember, natural make-up doesn't have to be invisible, but invisible make-up is beautiful too.**

Make-up must-haves for your handbag

Girls, as we know, our handbags are a complete must-have when we head out for the evening. How else would we carry the masses of things we seem to lug around everywhere with us? Have you ever emptied your handbag only to realise that you've been carrying around half of your bedroom's contents? I know I have. It seems to be every girl's prerogative to own a cavernous Mary Poppins bag! Well, we never know when we're going to need that little important something, and you can guarantee that if you leave it at home, you're going to want it.

So, just to make life a little bit simpler, here's a make-up must-have checklist for your handbag ...

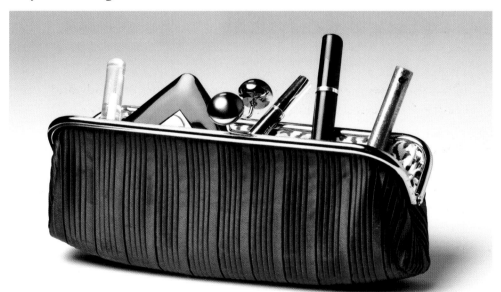

Lipstick

Lip gloss

Mascara

Eyeliner

Cover-up stick

Powder

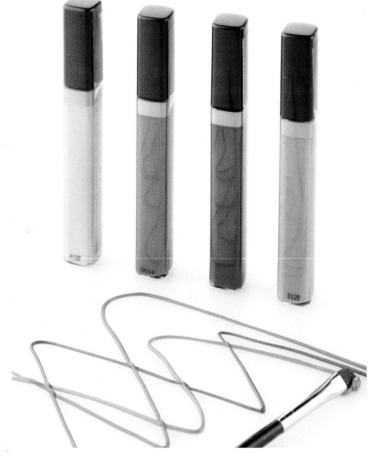

You honestly don't need to lug around your eyeshadows, foundation, blusher or bronzer. If you have used eye primer before applying your eyeshadow, and face primer beneath your foundation, and applied it properly, your make-up will stay put all night long.

CHAPTER 11

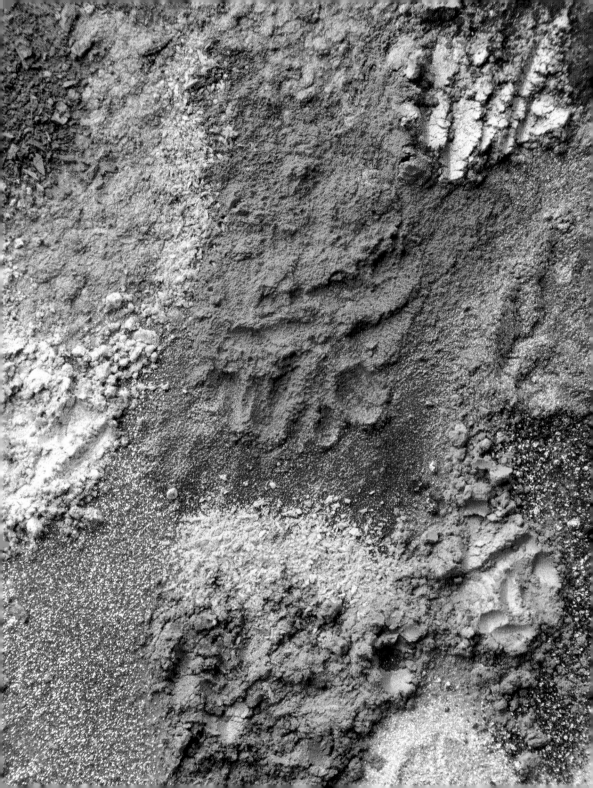

5-Minute Looks You'll Love

So I've shown you lots of techniques to help you apply your make-up successfully, but maybe you're thinking, how am I going to have time in the morning to get so technical?

In this section I've put together a selection of looks that you really can achieve in 5 minutes once you've mastered the art. They're simple, subtle, but striking. Keep practising and you'll be a pro in no time!

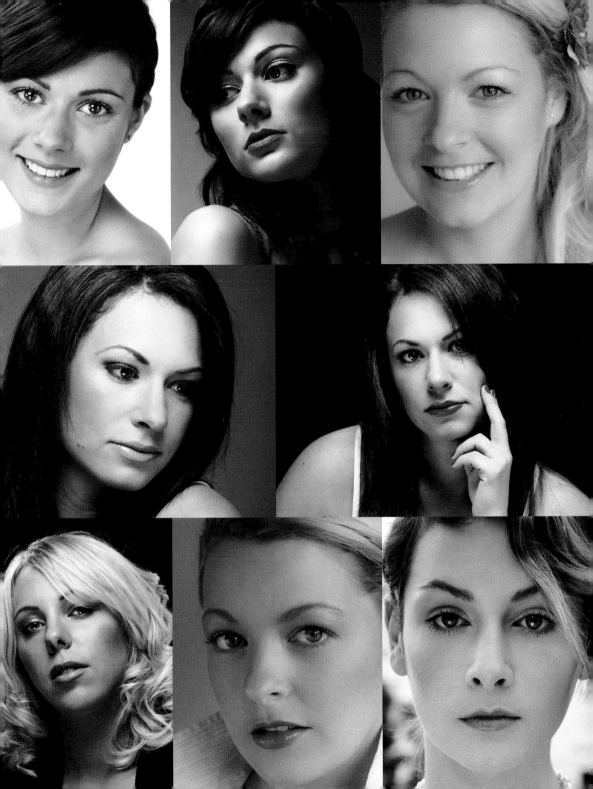

A flick of colour

A flick of coloured eye shadow and you've gone from bare face to bright and right on trend. It doesn't matter what time of year it is, this look never fails to give your outfit a zing. Switch your colours around to suit the season: try pastels for spring, brights for summer, bronzes for autumn and silvers for winter!

- Apply foundation primer to your face followed by foundation or tinted moisturiser if you desire.

- Pop some bronzer onto the apples of your cheeks, followed by a swish of apricot or pink blusher.

- Apply cream highlighter or a skin-toned eye shadow to your eyelids up to your brow bone and finish by patting turquoise eye shadow all over your eyelid stopping at the crease of your eyes.

- Blend any hard lines away. Apply mascara, and a nude lipstick. You're ready to hit the catwalk!

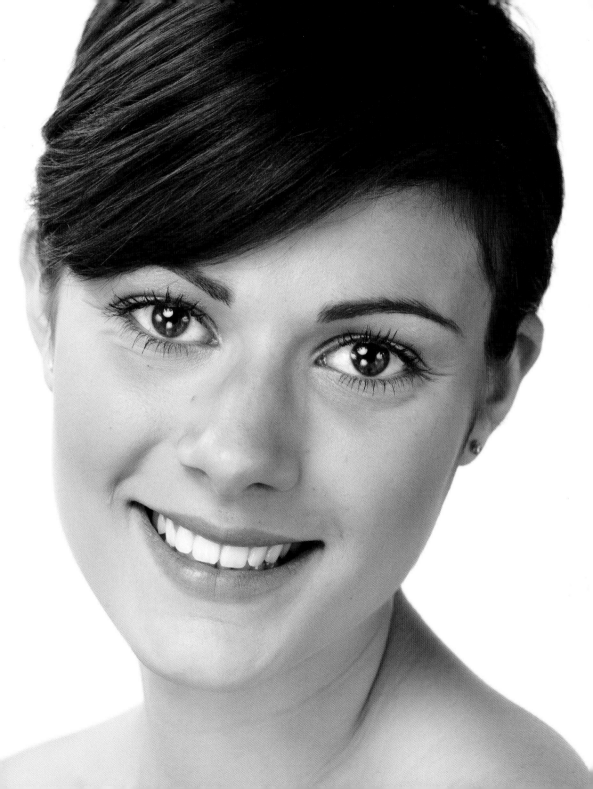

The ultimate glow

This look suits all seasons. In the summer it reflects the bright colours of the warm, golden weather; in the autumn it reflects the fiery colours of the falling leaves; in the winter it warms the world around you; and in the spring it reflects the fresh look of dewy flowers.

You could experiment with different coloured lipsticks to suit the seasons too. Peach for spring, coral for summer, orange for autumn and red for winter. You could even try glossy eyes for spring and summer and matt eyes for autumn and winter.

- Apply foundation primer to your face using the same technique as you use when putting on your moisturiser.

- Next use a tinted moisturiser or a very sheer cover foundation to give your skin a flawless glow that looks healthy and not over done.

- Your aim is flushed dewy skin, bronzed yet fresh. Pat an apricot cream blush into the apples of your cheeks and blend it up towards your temples.

- Dust your face with powder. Pop bronzer on your cheeks, forehead, nose, chin, and neck to give you a sun kissed glow.

- Dust shimmer across your eyes. The trick here is very simple fresh eyes, defined with a strong brow.

- Dust powder through your brows, a lighter brown at the beginning, darker towards the outer edges to give them a perfect shape that still looks natural and not over done. Finish with a fine coat of mascara.

- Give your look the ultimate glow with bright orange or coral lips.

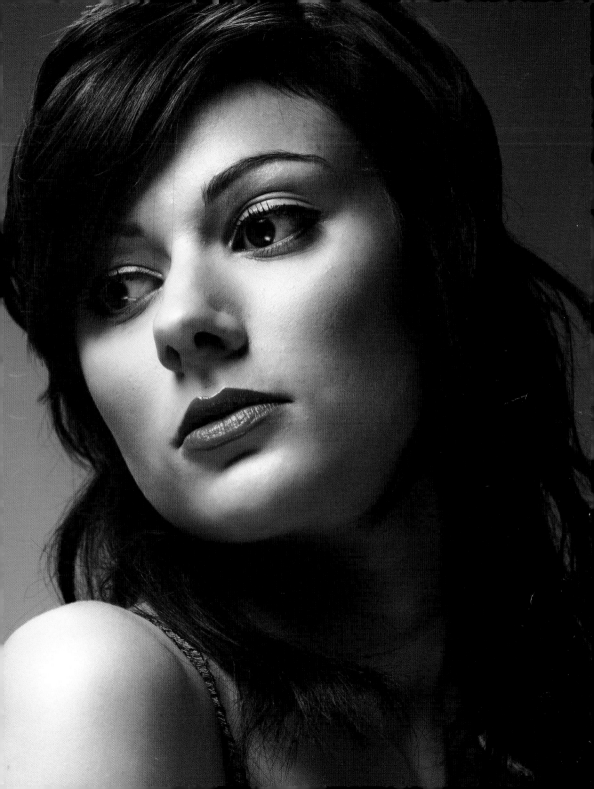

Pretty in pink

Soft flushed skin, subtle soft pink eyes and pretty pouty lips is a look that is beautiful no matter where you are or what you are doing. For a night on the town you look fresh faced and naturally pretty, guaranteed to make the guys melt! Yes it really is true that most men prefer natural, because it's real. They see the real you right from the start, with no hidden surprises, and lets face it who couldn't resist such an innocently pretty face! At work it's understated but professional and smart. At the beach it's lightweight, perfect for sunbathing and swimming - say goodbye to huge black panda eyes as you step out of the water!

Our model Jo's look reflects natural beauty perfectly. Here's how you can reflect yours too…

Prime your skin with foundation primer.

Buff a lightweight sheer foundation or tinted moisturiser into the areas of your face that you'd like to, whether it is all over your skin or in small areas.

Dust your face with a translucent powder to take away any stickiness, giving you soft, smooth skin ready for blush.

Brush some baby pink blusher onto the apples of your cheeks and blend it up towards your hairline.

Pop eye primer onto your eyes and blend it up to your brow bone.

Pat a baby pink eye shadow over your eyelids, stopping at the crease and blend any hard lines away.

Use your finger to dab a baby pink lipstick onto your lips, followed by a clear or baby pink lip-gloss for a flirty, glistening shine.

Simple smudged eyes

This look uses nude skin, nude lips and subtle, smudged eyes. It's not too dissimilar to the smokey eye, but is a little more understated than the big dark shadow you see on traditional smokey eyes.

If you are going all out on glamorous hair and clothes it's a good idea to keep the overall look simple rather than fussy, with too much detail.

This look emphasises features nicely and is great if you want a natural look with a bit of oomph.

- A soft, matt, bronzed complexion really flatters this look. After applying your primer and foundation, dust your skin with a translucent powder.

- Brush bronzer on all areas of your face that the sun kisses, your cheeks, forehead, nose, chin and neck. Make sure that you blend everything seamlessly so that there are no lines.

- Pop an apricot blusher onto the apples of your cheeks.

- Prime your eyes with eye primer and sweep a matt skin-toned shadow all over your eyelids up to your brow bone.

- Line your top lid with easy-smudge black kohl liner. Using a soft eye shadow brush, blend the liner all over your eyelid (no further than the crease).

- Smudge the black kohl liner along your bottom lash line and inside the inner rim if you would like to add more drama.

- Curl your lashes with eyelash curlers and sweep mascara from root to tip of your lashes top and bottom. Apply a second coat for more depth.

- Your eyes are the focus here, keep your lips nude with a skin-toned or pale shimmer lipstick or gloss. A clear pink lip-gloss also looks lovely.

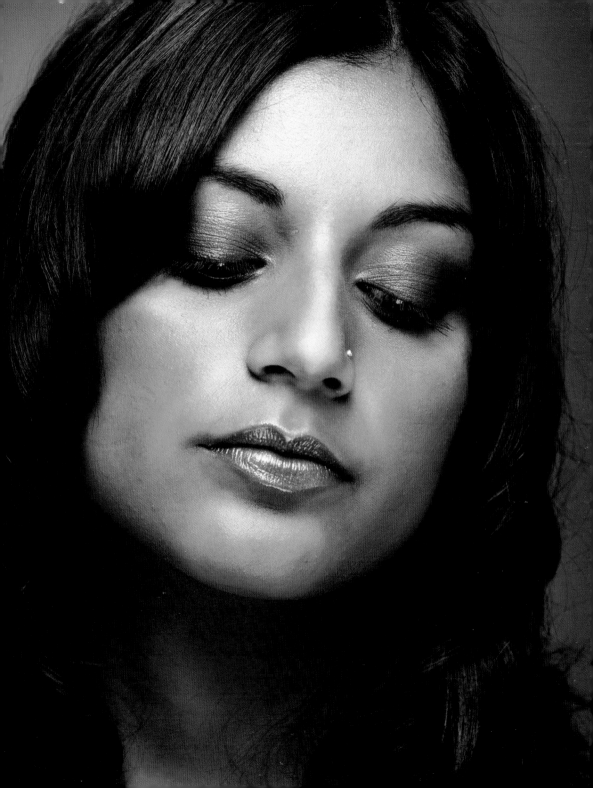

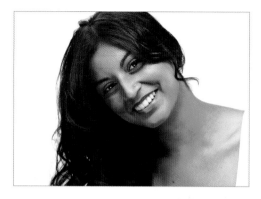
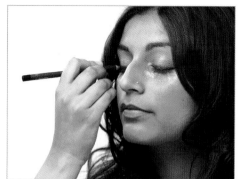
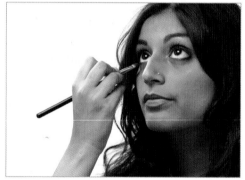
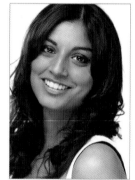

Turn simple smudged eyes into glam evening eyes using an irridescent purple shadow. Using your finger pat the irridescent shadow over the eyeliner to give the illusion of a shimmer of colour.

Apply a slight pink to your lips to make the colours pop.

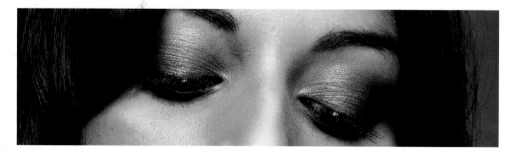

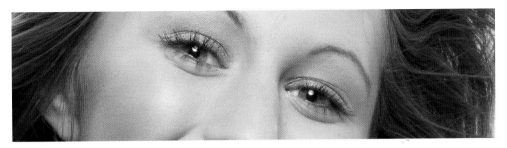

Simple smoky eyes

This smoky eye look is such a simple one to achieve. Whether your skin is dewy or matt, bronzed or English rose it will look gorgeous.

The trick is to apply an eye shadow slightly darker than your natural skin tone to your eyelids and blend it into the crease of your eyes until it fades into nothing near your brow bone. Smudge the same colour along your bottom lash line and apply mascara. Easy!

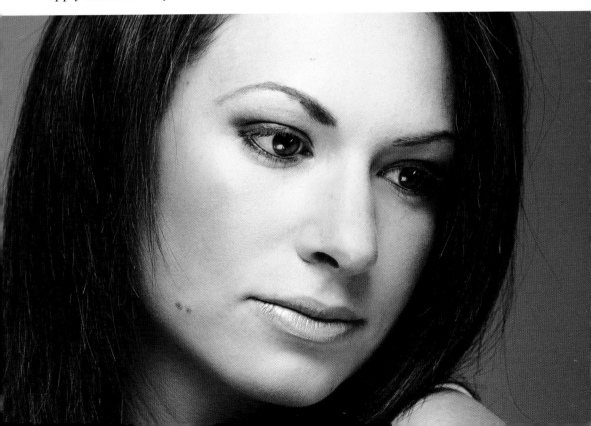

Mix n match

This look was inspired by the summer catwalk trends. Pops of colour on eyes and lips really light up the face and make a simple outfit really come to life.

Taking colour from your lid to the brow bone is brave and bold, but right on trend and very pretty.

Catwalk clothes are extremely dramatic; the idea behind them is for designers to display the full extent of their creativity. High street manufacturers then take elements of these designs and create more affordable, and easy-to-wear versions.

The same thing is done with make-up, I can show you how to take a really bold look and tone it down for everyday or party wear.

This look worn by model Jo, is very simple to re-create.

☐ Use a sheer purple shadow and dust it all over your eyelids and up to your brow bone.

☐ Keep your lower lash line free from eye shadow. Wearing eye shadow up to your brow bone is a big emphasis in itself, taking it underneath takes it too a really dramatic level. Have fun experimenting.

☐ Taking into consideration the theme of 'mix n match', I added coral lips for a twist. Whilst wearing colours that match looks lovely, the modern trends tell us that pretty much anything goes - there are no longer any boundaries where colour is concerned. So have some fun!

☐ Keep your skin soft and matt with this look, too much shine will confuse things, your eyes won't know where to look first. The focus should be cast upon your eyes and lips. Keep your cheeks subtle, give them a hint of a glow with a very light sweep of apricot blush.

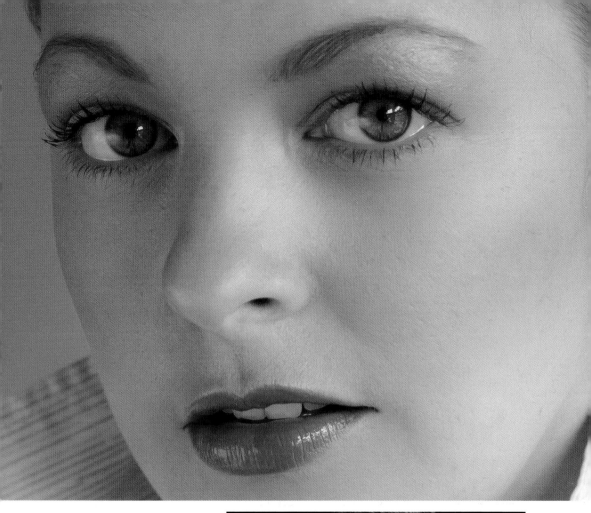

Go from day to night with simple eyes by adding deep pink lips and painting your nails bright orange. You can mix and match any colours to gain the same effect. An ultra modern look…

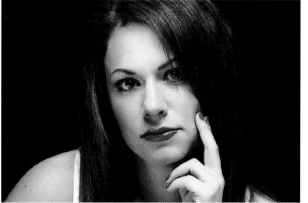

Gorgeous in gold

Here is another look that looks beautiful no matter what the season. It is natural yet warm, reflecting the colours of a summer's day. My inspiration behind this look is just that, the summer: Golden fields of corn and rays of sunshine glistening throughout the world and making everything beautiful. Bronze colours can be seen everywhere during the summer – in make-up, jewellery and clothes..

Our model Jes has fabulous blonde hair, which when put under the studio light lit up like the evening sun, highlighting her face. Have you ever noticed that the evening sun is the most flattering time of day? The golden tones of the setting sun soften our features. This is what I chose to recreate with Jes.
It may look complicated, but this look is really easy to achieve.

Apply your foundation primer followed by a sheer cover foundation or a tinted moisturiser.

Keep your skin dewy without being over-shiney by applying translucent powder to your t-zone, leaving your cheeks to glisten.

Contour your face with a matt bronzer emphasising your cheek bones and the areas where the sunlight would tan you naturally. Highlighting and shading is the trick to this look because it mimics the way the natural sunlight would play upon your face.

Apply eye primer to your eyelids and pat a gold metallic eye shadow over your eyelids.

Sweep a bronze shadow into the crease of your eyelids and blend it until there are no hard lines.

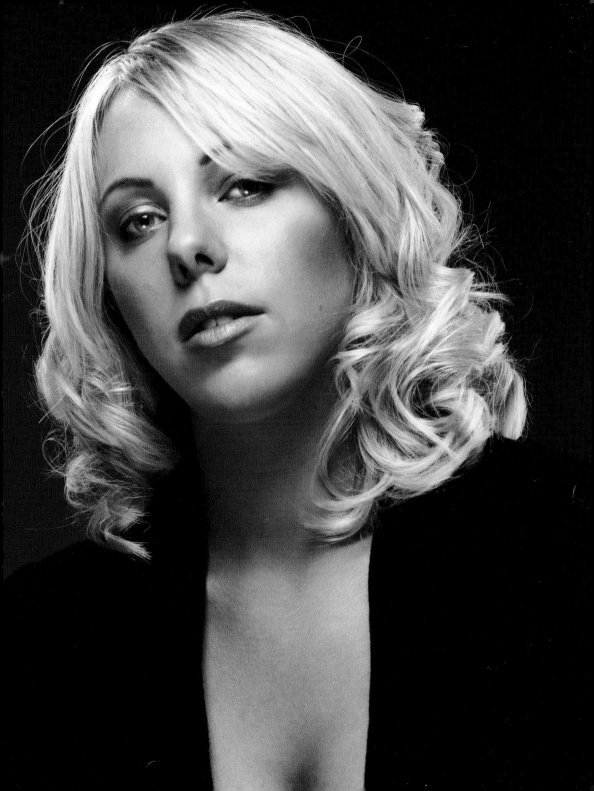

Office to evening...

Friday after work, after the last day of the week before the weekend and its time to unwind with friends …

Most people tend to head straight out from work on a Friday, but as we know corporate wear and leisure wear are completely different. However, it's really easy to turn your simple day-time make-up into a fun evening look – just add a dash of colour, a pop of blusher and a sweep of gloss and you're ready to go! Here's how to do it …

- Freshen your foundation up with a dust of translucent powder, pop a pinky blush onto the apples of your cheeks and blend it up towards your temples.

- Sweep a lilac shadow over your eyelids and blend it into the crease of your eyes.

- Sweep a turquoise shadow along your lower lash line.

- Apply eyeliner to the roots of your top lashes, followed by two coats of mascara.

- Finish the look with a nude pink lipstick.

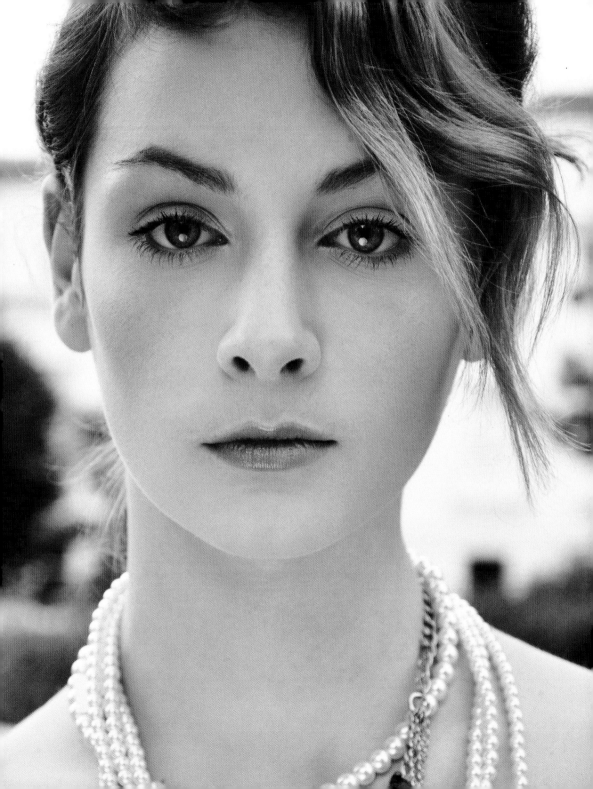

Simply natural

There are a million and one looks that we could create with make-up, but sometimes it's lovely just to look simply natural. Everyone's idea of what a natural look is with make-up is different - to some people even eye shadow feels too much. Here's an ultra simple look that looks fresh and gorgeous and is super quick, great for a work day morning!

☐ Apply foundation primer all over your face followed by your foundation.

☐ Dust your T Zone with translucent powder.

☐ Warm your skin with a little bronzer, sweep it beneath your cheeks, over your forehead, nose, chin and neck. Blend seamlessly.

☐ Pop some pinky peach blusher onto the apples of your cheeks.

☐ Apply mascara to your top and bottom lashes.

☐ Finish with a nude lipstick.

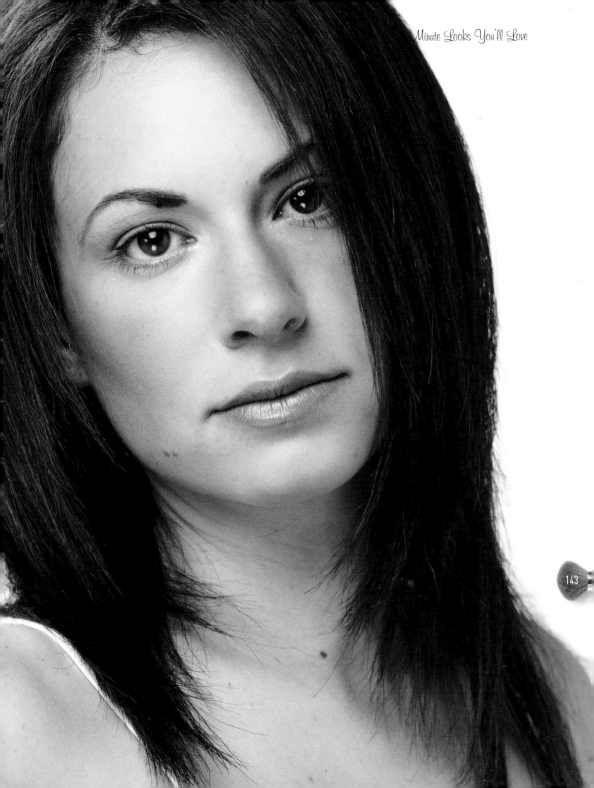

143

CHAPTER 12

Top Tips for Summer Skin...

◻ If you are happy with your skin, use an instant tan (wash off) or a semi permanent fake tan on your face rather than foundation. It is as light as a feather and looks radiant at all times! Its super quick to make-up too! Just add mascara and lip-gloss!

◻ If you need to take your foundation a shade darker to match your tan, mix it with an instant tan to create your perfect shade! As our tans tend to build gradually throughout the summer months, this enables you to darken your foundation gradually with it. Buying several different shades would become expensive and you may not be able to match your tan exactly as quickly as you can buy new shades. Fake tan has a yellow undertone, so whichever product you choose to mix with your foundation to make it darker, whether it be an instant tan or a darker shade of foundation, must contain yellow undertones too. Pink undertones will look unnatural next to a fake tan.

◻ During the summer your skin gets oily quickly, which absorbs more dirt from the surrounding air, keep up to speed on cleansing at night and remember to keep your pores clear by using a gentle face exfoliant once a week. Moisturise at night but keep it light in the morning.

Although your skin gets oily during the hot weather, it does not necessarily mean that it is hydrated, remember that in the beginning of this book I told you that if our skin gets too dry it would produce more oil. Drinking plenty of water will help to keep the pH balance of your skin more neutral and your body and skin hydrated, giving you even more of an ultimate glow.

If it's a hot day, try not wiping your face with your hands when your skin feels greasy or sweaty. Any bacteria on your hands will be transferred to your skin, which may cause spots!

When you head out to buy your sun screen for the summer, opt for a non-oily one on your face to prevent excess build up of grease on the surface of your skin, which could cause breakouts.

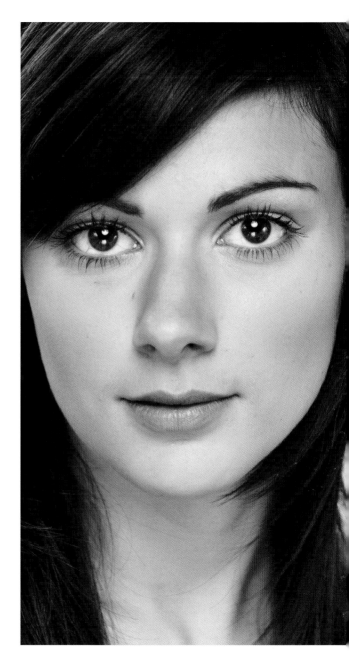

CHAPTER 13

Top Tips for Winter Skin...

The winter months are tough for our sensitive skin. The constant change in temperature, central heating and air conditioning really takes its toll. It's very important to protect our skin during these cold conditions, which really dehydrate and tighten our skin. The effect of this can make it feel sore and blotchy, so its very important to keep a brilliant beauty routine during this period.

- Cleanse your skin well but do not over cleanse. Cleansing at night will suffice, followed by a lovely thick, nourishing moisturiser over night to really feed and hydrate your skin whilst you are sleeping.

- If you have any extra dry areas you could use a vitamin E oil to replenish those areas.

- Use a nourishing facemask once a week.

- Use a rich body cream like body butter to help to keep the rest of your skin healthy.

- Remember your lips are very thin; they chap really easily so wear a moisturizing lip balm. Olive oil at night is fab and totally natural!

During the winter because it is colder we often feel less thirsty, remember not to neglect your body, drink plenty of water to keep your body hydrated, a lack of water is a common reason for dry skin alongside the cold weather.

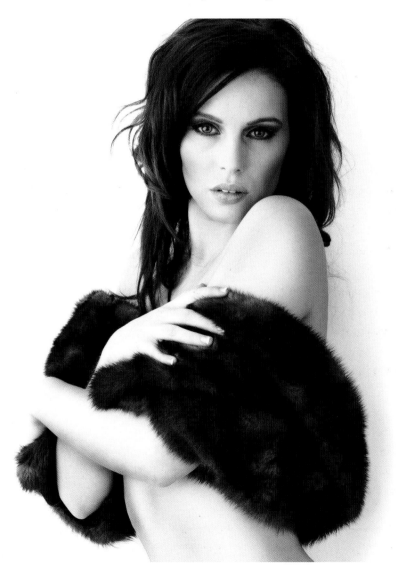

CHAPTER 14

The Beauty of Nature

Why natural is fabulous

The word natural is heard everywhere today. Being natural is becoming important for many areas of our lives, whether it's food, cosmetics or clothing.

When I shop for food, I try to opt for organic or free-range foods, which means that they are grown naturally without the use of pesticides. Eating well does wonders for our bodies, helping to keep us healthy and radiant. Consider how you feel after you've binged on fatty foods. Do you feel lethargic? Does your skin feel less radiant? Do you get breakouts? These are common side effects of a poor diet. On the other hand, when we eat a good balanced diet, containing plenty of water, veg, fruit, and very little sugar we tend to feel energetic and beautiful.

However, taking care of your body doesn't mean that you can't eat the occasional yummy treat. You can! I've grown up with the attitude that although too much of something is never good, a little of what you fancy doesn't hurt. So, next time you reach for that chocolate cake, think 'one slice will make a nice treat but that's all I need'.

The same perspective applies to the world of skin care. We are all guilty of heading to bed without taking our make-up off from time to time, and I for one should know better. But the odd slip doesn't hurt as long as we skip back into a healthy routine.

What we put onto our skin has the same effect as our diet. Natural products nourish and care for our skin, whilst synthetic products can make our skin feel dull.

What makes a product natural?

A natural product is a product that contains ingredients that are plant derived. There are many products on the market with labels reading 100% natural, but unfortunately this is not always as true as it reads. People assume that because a product is natural it will be organic, however the same rules apply here as they do to food. Carrots are natural, because they are plants, but some carrots are organic because they are grown without the help of any chemicals, other carrots are not organic because they are grown with the use of pesticides etc. This is the same with our cosmetics. If you read the ingredients on the label you may find that many other chemicals have been used in order to increase the product's shelf life. It is possible to find products that are 100% natural and organic but you need to get savvy!

Keep in mind that products can contain less than 5% natural ingredients to be called a natural product. All natural means 100%! That's a huge margin of difference.

What are the benefits of using a natural product?

Natural products are gentle to our skin and often contain medicinal properties that help to fight skin conditions such as acne rosecea and spots. For example mineral make-up is non-comedogenic, this means that it allows your skin to breathe without blocking your pores. There are many mineral make-ups on the market, some better than others. Watch out for products containing talc, talc is the most aging product you can put on your skin!

> Switch your standard powder to a mineral powder for a talc free option.

Synthetic products are man-made and can therefore contain harsh chemicals. These are often hypoallergenic causing sensitised skin and the product blocks the pores reducing the amount that our skin is able to breathe, which in turn can lead to a break out of spots. There are so many natural products on the market that you don't need to use synthetic ones. And natural products are much friendlier to our environment.

Our skin absorbs anything we put onto it; which means that if we put chemicals onto our skin, we are absorbing toxins. Natural products on the other hand feed our skin as they are absorbed.

Natural products are generally more expensive, because they cost more to make. Plant derived products need to be stabilized in order for them to last. Synthetic products are cheap because chemicals are much easier to mass-produce.

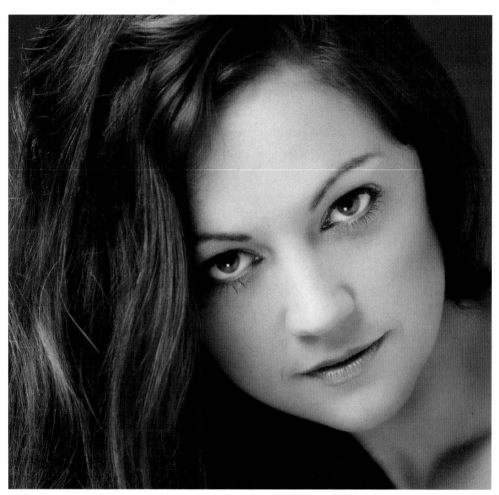

CHAPTER 15

Aloe Vera — Nature's Gift

Aloe Vera is one of nature's most incredible products. In this chapter, Anne Blackwood, our Aloe Vera expert explains the benefits of this miracle plant.

The Miracle Plant Explained

Aloe Vera is known by lots of different names around the world, the most well-known being Miracle Plant, Burn Plant, Nature's Healer, First Aid Plant, Silent Healer. The Japanese have a name for it which means 'no need for a doctor'.

It has been used for thousands of years, with the ancient Egyptians first understanding its benefits to the skin.. Two of the most famous Egyptian queens – Cleopatra and Nefertiti are thought to have used Aloe Vera as a part of their beauty regime. There are lots of pictures of Aloe Vera in the Pharaohs' tombs, and it was regularly used by the ancient Egyptians for medicinal purposes as well as for skin beauty.

For centuries it was used medicinally by many people around the world, particularly in the hot countries where it grew naturally. With the discovery of antibiotics in the early 1900s the focus for medicine switched from herbal remedies to manufactured drugs. Recently, with the problem of resistance to antibiotics causing great concern and renewed interest in natural remedies, the health benefits of Aloe Vera have been taken seriously again.

What is Aloe Vera?

Aloe Vera (translated as True Aloe) looks like a cactus, but is actually a member of the lily family and is a type of plant known as a succulent. There are over 200 different types of Aloe plants, but only five have medicinal properties, of these Aloe Vera is by far the most potent.

The Aloe likes hot dry climates and has a tough outer skin which is designed to keep the moisture in. Inside the leaf is a thick squishy gel which contains the beneficial properties. This gel has lots of fantastic properties which will help your skin through those challenges that are often experienced in the teenage years and early 20s, such as a spotty skin, (including acne), and dry patches. It also helps relieve itchy skin problems such as eczema and psoriasis too.

How Aloe Vera works

The dermis is the skin layer where new skin cells are produced, and the skin needs nourishment to renew, grow and develop new healthy cells. Aloe is unique in its ability to penetrate the skin to the dermis level without the aid of synthetic substances. A product, which is made using a high percentage of Aloe Vera inner gel, will penetrate seven layers of skin tissue, compared with many creams that can only manage two. This means that healing is from the inside out, without producing a surface that is greasy and attracts dirt and bacteria. It is then able to help repair tissue quickly and with minimal scarring.

This is very important, since the skin is a very efficient organ for absorption (think of contraceptive and nicotine patches), and about 60% of anything you put on your skin will be absorbed into your body.

Aloe moisturises by binding moisture into the tissues without sealing the skin and allowing oxygen to reach the skin so it can breathe properly. This is another very important part of the healing process and keeping skin in healthy condition.

Many of the cheaper creams and lotions will seal the skin making bacterial and fungal infections much more likely. There is nothing these infections like more, than a warm, damp environment, which is what is created when the skin is sealed.

Benefits of Aloe Vera

Aloe has the same pH factor as human skin (4.5 – 5.5) which is also vital for healthy skin, and is naturally hypoallergenic. It naturally adapts to each individual skin type so is suitable for greasy, combination and dry skins.

Aloe is a natural cleanser and has antibiotic, antiviral and antifungal properties so will help to reduce the effects of skin infections. It also is very good at softening hard skin.

Scientific tests have proved that Aloe accelerates the rate of healing by up to 35% and, combined with its antibiotic properties, it reduces the chance of scarring. Its heat-reducing and anti-inflammatory properties will make swollen and painful skin feel more comfortable and help with the healing process.

When Aloe Vera is combined with other substances to make skin creams, it helps all of these additives work much better in improving the skin's condition.

As well as keeping the skin moisturised to protect from dryness and flaking skin, it will also help protect from insect bites as it is a natural insect repellant.

Aloe is not known as the Burn Plant for nothing – it is excellent for treating burns – including sunburn.

The small size of its molecules means it is absorbed into the skin very quickly so you have its benefits without having a greasy slippery skin after application, unlike many creams and lotions.

Aloe Vera and its extremely beneficial properties make it ideal to use for a basis of a good complexion and encourages good health both inside and out.

Because Aloe is able to adapt to each skin type it is suitable for anyone.

153

Aloe helps to Keep you Safe in the Sun

Aloe is very good at helping to protect the skin, and if it is the main ingredient, it is beneficial in sunscreen lotions.

Recent research has shown that lots of people still don't realise that sunshine can seriously damage the skin, and over the years excessive exposure can lead to skin cancer. Using a good quality protective sunscreen can reduce that risk significantly. When in the sun it is essential to use a lotion that has an SPF of 30 or more to give the skin good protection from the damaging effects of the sun.

An SPF value is the length of time you can stay in the sun covered with sunscreen compared to unprotected skin. For example, an SPF of 30 means your skin will take 30 times longer to burn than if you were unprotected, and it will almost completely protect you against harmful ultraviolet rays.

UVA & UVB RAYS explained

The two harmful rays from the sun are known as UVA (Ultra Violet A) and UVB (Ultra Violet B).

UVA ages the skin and penetrates deeply. This is the one that causes the skin to tan, but it is worth knowing that tanning is the skin's way of trying to protect itself against damage. A tanned skin can look good, but it's your skin's way of telling you it has a problem and is not happy.

UVB burns and is responsible for sunburn and redness. Excessive exposure to sun over the years will damage the skin cells and could cause cancer.

Using sunscreen doesn't mean you can stay out in the sun longer than is sensible, but it does reduce the chances of skin damage. The best sunscreens will protect against both UVA and UVB rays.

The Victorians had the right idea when they avoided the sun and regarded tanned skins in ladies as socially unacceptable; although since we need vitamin D for healthy bones, we should have about 15 minutes of sun on our skin two to three times a week to produce that vitamin naturally. (This time depends on the colour of your skin and whether the sun is strong or weak). Dark skins need longer in the sun than fair skins and the sun must be on skin without sunscreen.

Introducing Aloe Vera into your skincare routine

Since beauty starts from the inside, and problems are best addressed at the source, the first thing to think about is drinking Aloe Vera (yes, you can drink it!).

To accompany the drink, look for skincare products, that are made primarily from Aloe Vera, in order to benefit the outside.

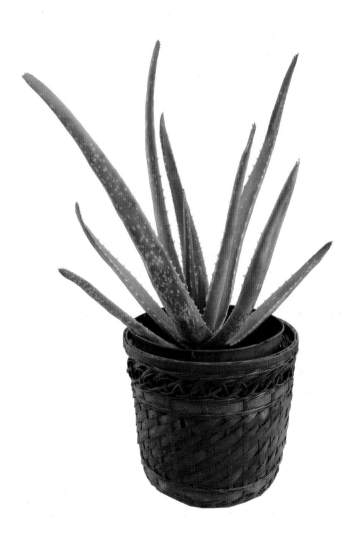

Aloe Vera as a Drink

First make sure you get the right Aloe drink.

The most effective drink is one that is made from the inner gel only, without the need to filter it. It then still contains all these fantastic benefits. Aloe drinks that are readily available from chemists and health shops on the high street tend to be made from the whole leaf, rather than from the inner gel.

The Aloe Science Council certifies the basic quality of Aloe products and for drinks it requires a minimum 15% content of Aloe to be awarded their logo. However for an Aloe Vera drink to be really effective you need 75% Aloe inner gel content.

Think of orange squash compared with freshly squeezed orange juice and you have an idea of the difference. If you wanted vitamin C would you drink orange squash? This is one of the main differences between whole leaf filtered drinks and those using only the inner gel.

So read your labels carefully as many companies will add Aloe Vera to their products and it will be listed somewhere near the bottom, which means that there is only a very small percentage of this fabulous plant in their products.

The best quality Aloe Vera drinks and skin creams are not really available on the high street. However there is a company who currently uses only the filleted inner gel of the leaf, with a high content of Aloe Vera in all of their products - both drinks and skincare products. Their drinks which contain up to 97% Aloe, are essentially the same as the contents of the inner gel, and their products are generally available through home-based businesses, and not currently on the high street. This same company also produces an excellent range of cosmetics based on Aloe Vera.

By using Aloe Vera and sourcing products that have the inner gel of the plant as their main ingredient, you can look after your skin in the best possible way, providing superior soothing, healing and moisturising qualities that occur naturally.

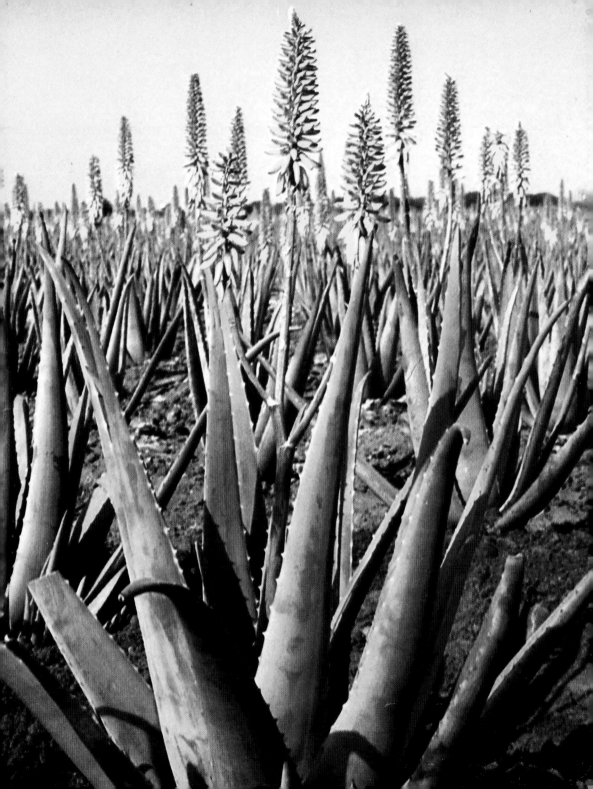

CHAPTER 16

Your Questions Answered

Is wearing foundation every day bad for my skin? What can I do if I want to let my skin have a day off but I don't want to go totally bare faced?

Wearing foundation every day is not bad for your skin if the foundation is of a good quality and contains natural ingredients. Even so it is good to let your skin breathe occasionally without it. Many women who I meet and who have amazing skin, actually don't often wear foundation.

Try having make-up free days and always take your make-up off when you go to bed. If your skin is going through a good cycle and you can go without foundation, pop a primer on your skin and dust bronzer and blusher on your cheeks to give you a glow.

If you simply can't bear the thought of not wearing anything on your skin, why not opt for a tinted moisturiser, or buff a light mineral foundation over your skin instead of thick a foundation.

Can I really sleep in mineral make-up?

There's a lot of hype about mineral make-up being so pure that you can sleep in it. I would never recommend sleeping in any of your make-up, no matter how pure and organic it is. Skin is most active at night and so should be given time to breathe, recover and be nourished. Night time is the time for a great moisturiser.

How can I make my make-up last all day?
I'm often asked how professionals are able to apply make-up that stays put all day long. There are occasions, such as when doing bridal make-up, when stay-put factor is super important! Well the secret is primer. I use foundation primer all over the face before applying foundation, and also I use an eye primer before eye shadow.

Does mineral foundation really have the same coverage as liquid foundations?
Completely! Remember, mineral foundation is not a powder, although it has the consistency of one it is in fact finely ground rocks (minerals) which when applied to the skin have an almost creamy texture. A tiny amount goes a long way; use your brush to buff the mineral into your skin using circular motions. You can build the coverage bit by bit.

Should we encourage or discourage young girls to experiment with make-up?
Regardless of what us mums say, our children will start experimenting with make-up at some point. In my opinion when my daughter reaches the age when she wants to experiment with make-up, rather than focusing on the negatives, I will teach her the right way to apply make-up for the age that she is.

I feel really low in confidence about the way I look, how can I feel more positive?
Try a new style out everyday, whether it be with your make-up, hair or clothes. This helps you to be creative and to *find a* look you *feel confident and comfortable with.*

My skin is really oily and my make-up slides off my face! Is there anything that I can do to help this?
Yes, if you use a moisturiser in the morning ensure that it is oil free. Next apply a foundation primer to your skin before your foundation, this will help to minimise the pores and soak up excess oil. Spray a fixing spray mist over your face once your foundation is applied, it makes your skin feel fresh and will give your make-up extra staying power. Keep a small pot of mineral powder in your handbag ready for touch ups if you need them, or my favourite Laura Mercier mattifying cream.

I love fake tan, but is it healthy for me to wear it continuously?
You can use a fake tan continuously. Fake tans are designed to work on the top layers of your skin, not to penetrate it. As always, check the ingredients in the product before you buy to ensure that you feel happy that what you are putting onto your skin is healthy.

I feel really self conscious about my body when I'm getting a spray tan and worry what the therapist might think of me, is this normal?
Everyone gets body conscious – no one feels perfect. So we're all in the same boat. I spray tan my clients regularly and I can honestly say that when I am carrying out the treatment, my focus is solely on the task in hand. I see the body as an art form, the curves of the body, the highlight and shadows of the skin and concentrate on getting the colour perfect. It is important during the treatment to keep conversation flowing, and you will feel relaxed and confident in no time.

I have really pale skin and would love to look bronzed, how do I choose the right shade?
Bronzer should only ever be a couple of shades darker than your natural skin tone, otherwise it looks unnatural. It should mimic the colour that you go when you have a real tan, so for very pale skin, use a bronzer with an apricot / peach undertone. Brown will look muddy.

What make-up colours make a tan pop?
Think about the colours that hit the shops during the summer months, these are the colours that will really complement your bronzed skin. Always opt for warm-toned colours during the summer months like bronze, peach, apricot, gold, turquoise, pinky purples, yellow and even warm greens. Anything goes as long as it doesn't look cold. Cold colours can make a tan look flat.

What colours should I opt for during the winter months?
During the winter, unless you have a spray tan, your skin is paler, so opt for cooler

toned colours. These will fit nicely with the season and complement cool skin. For girls with darker skin tones try silvers and blues and deep purples as a great winter colour.

I get really dark under-eyes, what is causing this?
Dark under-eyes can mean a number of things. Sometimes it is hereditary, in that the pigment in our skin is different from person to person so some people are born with pigmentation patches, others may develop them over time. It's all down to genes.

However, if dark under-eyes is something that you suffer from only now and again, the chances are it could have something to do with your diet. Are you eating enough water- based foods, such as fruit and veg? Dehydration can be another cause of dark under eyes because the skin is so thin there. Try drinking lots of water and see what happens. The other reason is a common one – lack of sleep. 8 hours a night is needed if possible to get your beauty sleep. If you are worried about it, contact your GP, as health issues can effect our skin.

CHAPTER 17

Be Inspired

Applying make-up is an art form. Every catwalk creation has been inspired by an object, or an emotion or a living thing. I recently saw some wonderful blue, green and gold eye make-up that had been inspired by peacocks.

Many great artists have inspired me throughout my journey as a make-up artist. As a make-up artist it is extremely important to keep up to date with all of the latest trends. When I work for a fashion designer the make-up theme always needs to follow, complement and reflect their ideas. For example, if the fashion is pastel florals, the make-up will generally be soft, feminine and pretty. A more military style of clothing would be teamed with a bolder more military style make-up, such as strong lips, brows and eyeliner.

When I meet a client and am asked to create a look for them, I take into account their clothing, hairstyle and colour, features and face shape first. I then form ideas from their personality: what do they like or dislike?

Why not try creating your own looks? Set yourself a challenge and see how many new looks you can create from the things that inspire you. This could be from an image you see in a magazine, some art work that you see, nature, people that you meet, even animals. Focus on things that you like and see where your imagination takes you! The following pages show some more great looks to inspire you. Have fun!

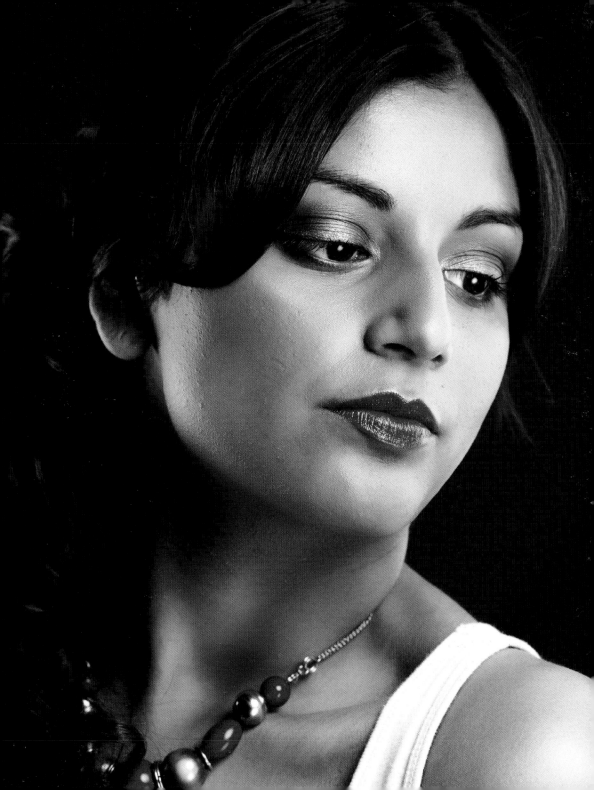

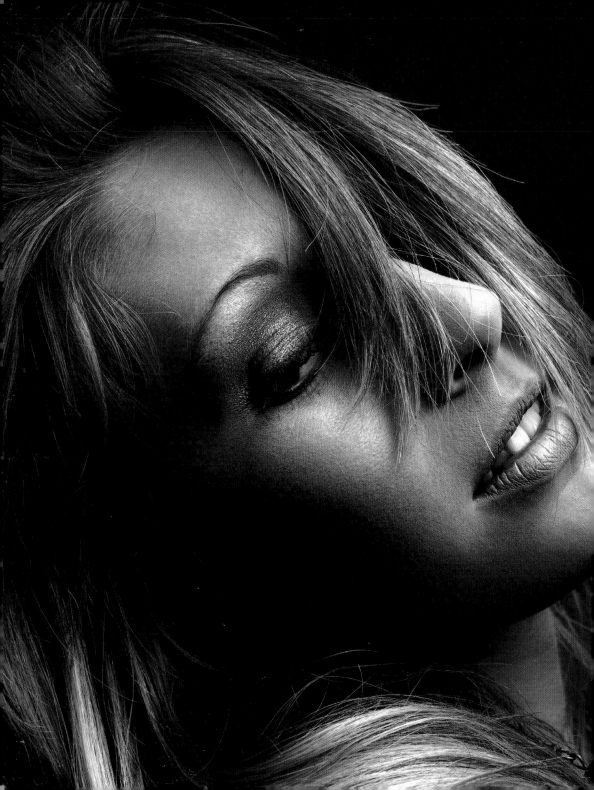

Acknowledgements

I would like to dedicate this book to every single girl in the world! I hope that my book not only teaches you to love yourself and your make-up, but also inspires you to work towards realising your own dreams, as I have realised mine.

My daughter Lara has been a huge inspiration behind the writing of this book. I hope that, in time, as she grows up, she too will use this guide and look up to me as a role model.

I would like to thank everyone who has been a part of my life throughout the process of this book coming together. Thanks to John at Waterham Studios for working so hard with me to create some amazing photographs for the book, and for being my great friend and mentor throughout my career as a make-up artist.

Jordan at Portal PR, meeting you led me to fulfil my dream of becoming a successful make-up artist and now an author. Thank you for every piece of advice and help that you have ever given me.

I would like to say a special thank you to all of the girls who have modelled for my book, and to everyone who has been part of the publishing process. Thanks to Natalie Shirlaw for your incredibly talented hair styling, for your time, and for your belief in me; to Marcello Pozetti at Prima Donna Studios for the fabulous photo of Beckie on page 12; and to Matt Roobol (www.mustardmatt.com) for your genius website design and marketing.

Thanks also to my family and friends for believing in me and supporting me every step of the way: to my dad Nic for your fabulous input within the book and for being a proud father; to my mum Christine for being 100% supportive from start to finish; to my sister Jess for all your lovely cups of tea and biscuits, and for your help on the photo shoots – in particular, the wind machine!

Thank you to Lucy, Rachel and Paula for making me feel bubbly, even through the tough times.

Thank you also to Nichola Joss for being my inspiration into make-up artistry and for supporting me with this book. (www.nicolajoss.com)

Finally, I would like to thank my partner Anton, for boosting my confidence sky high and for filling me with happiness.

I hope you have all enjoyed reading my book as much as I have enjoyed writing it.

Photographers

John Burgess has contributed the majority of photographs in this book, but I'd also like to thank the following photographers for also contributing photographs.

John Burgess – www.waterhamphotographicstudios.co.uk
All photos other than those specifically credited below.

Lotte Simons Photography – pages 9, 10 and 141 www.lottesimons.com

Ben Anker Photography – pages 2 and 164 www.benankerphotography.co.uk

Samantha Jones Photography – pages 131 and 137 (top image) www.samanthajonesphotography.co.uk

Marcello Pozzetti – page 12 www.primadonna.org.uk

Giant Arc Design – Colour chart on page 38 www.giantarc.co.uk

Charles Blackwood – Pages 155 and 157

Models

Bethany Rose – front cover, pages 20, 56, 94-97 and 100

Florence West – pages 107 and 117

Minnie Rahman – pages 133, 134 and 163

Lucie Vigar – pages 18, 21, 35 and 43

Chloe Rees – page 109

Hannah Foster – page 115

Katherine – page 119

Nichola Mayall – page 102 www.TiarasAndFascinators.com

Hayley O'Connell-White – pages 2, 48-55, 58, 62-67, 70, 84, 88, 90 and 111

Colour – pages 15, 26, 33, 39, 68 and 79

Kirsty Hicks – page 147

Laura Masters – pages 83 and 87

Emily Nel – page 104

Rebecca Richardson – page 12

Natalie Perie – pages 77 and 106

Aviva Stone – pages 135, 137 (second image) and 143

Sophia Pittounikos – pages 127, 129 and 145

Sophie Godliman – pages 9, 10 and 141 www.shinemodelmanagement.com

Sarah Reeves – page 150

Jes Braithwaite – pages 28 and 139

Jo Baigent– pages 131 and 137 (first image)

Expert advice

Anne Blackwood

Aloe Vera Expert

Chapter 15, pages 151–157

Index

Healing Foods, Healthy Foods
Use superfoods to help fight disease and maintain a
healthy body

Gloria Halim

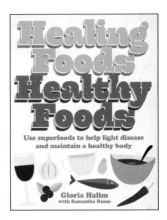

Cutting out processed and junk foods from your diet and
introducing the superfoods listed in this book can help you
to boost your immune system and increase your energy
levels. Superfoods are rich in vitamins, minerals and anti-
oxidants. This book lists them individually and explains
why they are so good for you and how they can help keep
you healthy.

It also lists a number of spices which have medicinal benefits in their own right. By
combining these spices with some of the superfoods, this book includes some simple but
delicious recipes that have their roots in the Mediterranean, Asian and African regions,
all of which are known for having the healthiest diets in the world.

There are mouthwatering salads, wholesome soups, delicious main courses and
vegetable dishes, fresh juices and nutritious smoothies.

You really are what you eat and with this book to guide you, you can change your eating
habits for the better and make a difference to your general health.

Author Gloria Halim changed her 'junk food' habits and followed the superfood route
after having gone through health problems. Since recovering she feels healthier and more
energetic than ever before. She has been helped in the writing of this book by Sami
Rosso, a graduate of The Institute of Optimum Nutrition, who has been working as a
nutritionist for ten years and advises the general public and athletes on their diets.

ISBN 978-1-905862-53-5

Make Your Own Perfume
How to create your own fragrances to suit mood,
character and lifestyle

Sally Hornsey

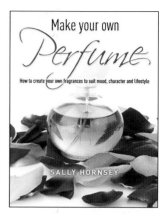

Wearing perfume is often limited by the cost of designer
brands. Blending your own fragrance takes perfume
wearing to another level. You can design your own perfume
to suit your mood, your character and your lifestyle – and,
of course, your budget!

Make Your Own Perfume guides you through individual aromas, showing you how to
design and structure perfume for yourself and for others. It sets out blending tips to help
you create your own range of gorgeous signature scents, fragrances that you can wear as
often as you like.

In this book you will discover how to:
- Identify the fragrance families and choose which ones are better suited to different
  occasions;
- Classify both natural and synthetic oils into 'note' categories to enable you to balance
  your perfume;
- Make tinctures and infusions to use in your perfumes;
- Dilute your perfume blend to become a body spray, eau de toilette, *eau de parfum*,
  pure perfume, or after shave;
- Package your perfume - and choose appropriate names for it;
- Create perfume blends for pot pourri, reed diffusers and other room scenting
  products.

Sally Hornsey runs *Plush Folly*, a private cosmetic training company, specialising in a
range of cosmetic-making workshops, kits, and home study courses. Sally's interest in
perfume began when she managed the perfume counter for a well-known department
store. Since then, her nose has taken Sally on a perfume adventure and she enjoys having
beautiful aromas and fragrances woven into her life. She has blended perfumes with
celebrities on the radio and on television, and created an aftershave with the England
Rugby team that actually smelt good!

ISBN 978-1-905862-69-6

Make Your Own Skincare Products

How to create skincare applications for particular skin types

Sally Hornsey

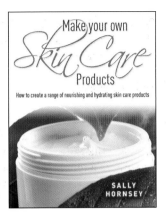

If treated and nourished properly your skin will be healthy and glowing, making you feel good and look great.

This book will guide you through creating your own personal range of skincare applications, tailored to your particular skin type – or anybody else's. The products made use natural ingredients where possible, and throughout the book you will find details of the purpose and benefits of the ingredients used. You will also learn about ingredients that can be substituted so that you can adapt the recipes to suit your or others' needs.

In this book you will discover how to:
- Choose essential oils that are useful for treating different skin conditions;
- Design and create a range of products including a cleanser, toner, face mask and moisturising cream;
- Identify the ingredients that are beneficial in hand-made skin care products;
- Make informed choices on which ingredients are most appropriate for different skin conditions;
- Make tinctures and infusions to use in your products;
- Store your products to ensure that they are fresh and safe to use.

Sally Hornsey runs *Plush Folly*, a private cosmetic training company, specialising in a range of cosmetic-making workshops, kits and home study courses. Sally has taught many students how to design a range of skin care products for their own use and has given students the skills and knowledge they need to establish a flourishing business.

ISBN 978-1-905862-68-9

The Step-by-Step Guide to Planning Your Wedding

Lynda Wright

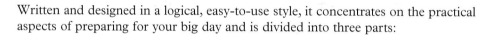

Your wedding day marks the beginning of a new and exciting chapter in your life, so you'll want to make sure it's as wonderful as you always dreamed it would be.

This book will guide you through all the organisational detail of your wedding preparations so that you'll feel completely confident about the many choices and decisions you will have to make.

Written and designed in a logical, easy-to-use style, it concentrates on the practical aspects of preparing for your big day and is divided into three parts:

- The Countdown Calendar, detailing all the vital steps at each stage of the preparations.

- The Action Plans, showing the step-by-step sequences needed to organise the transport, flowers, photography and all the other essentials.

- The Checklists, providing lots of space for you to record all the relevant information, so that you can track your progress and ensure that nothing has been overlooked.

If you follow this book step by step, you'll feel confident that your big day will be a wonderful success and one that you'll remember for the rest of your life.

ISBN 978-1-84528-410-7

Exploring Your Dreams
How to use dreams for personal growth and creative inspiration

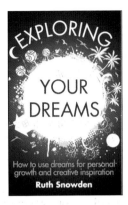

Ruth Snowden

Dreams are an integral part of who we are and carry valuable messages. They can reveal our true selves, unmasking our fears, hostilities, hidden talents and desires. Enabling us to explore and learn from hidden aspects of the psyche, dreams can teach you a lot about yourself and others, helping you with problems and guiding you throughout your life.

This book gives advice and guidance on exploring and interpreting your dreams, and using them for personal and creative development. It includes:

- The place of dreams in human culture
- How to prepare for, and how to record your dreams
- Dream analysis, including common dream types and the strange but powerful world of symbolism
- Advanced dream exploration, including joining a dream group and working with others.

ISBN 978-1-84528-466-4

How To Books are available through all good bookshops,
or you can order direct from us through Grantham Book Services.

Tel: +44 (0)1476 541080
Fax: +44 (0)1476 541061
Email: orders@gbs.tbs-ltd.co.uk
or via our website: www.howtobooks.co.uk

To order via any of these methods please quote the title(s) of the book(s) and your
credit card number together with its expiry date.

For further information about our books and catalogue, please contact:
How To Books, Spring Hill House, Spring Hill Road, Begbroke, Oxford OX5 1RX

Visit our web site at: www.howtobooks.co.uk
or you can contact us by email at
info@howtobooks.co.uk